CW01558673

The Acid Reflux Diet Cookbook for Beginners

1800 Days of Healthy, Easy & Delicious Recipes to Help Relieve Heartburn & Reduce Discomfort. Includes a 28-Day Meal Plan for Managing GERD & LPR Symptoms

Amanda Ray

© Copyright 2025 - All rights reserved.

The content contained within this book may not be reproduced, duplicated, or transmitted without direct written permission from the author or publisher. Under no circumstances will any blame or legal responsibility be held against the publisher or author for any damages, reparations, or monetary losses due to the information contained within this book, either directly or indirectly.

<u>Legal Notice:</u>

This book is copyright-protected. It is only for personal use. You cannot amend, distribute, sell, use, quote, or paraphrase any part of the content within it without the consent of the author or publisher.

<u>Disclaimer Notice:</u>

Please note that the information contained within this document is for educational and entertainment purposes only. All efforts have been made to present accurate, up-to-date, reliable, and complete information. No warranties of any kind are declared or implied. Readers acknowledge that the author does not render legal, financial, medical, or professional advice. The content within this book has been derived from various sources. Please consult a licensed professional before attempting any techniques outlined in this book.

By reading this document, the reader agrees that under no circumstances is the author responsible for any direct or indirect losses incurred as a result of the use of the information contained within this document, including, but not limited to, errors, omissions, or inaccuracies.

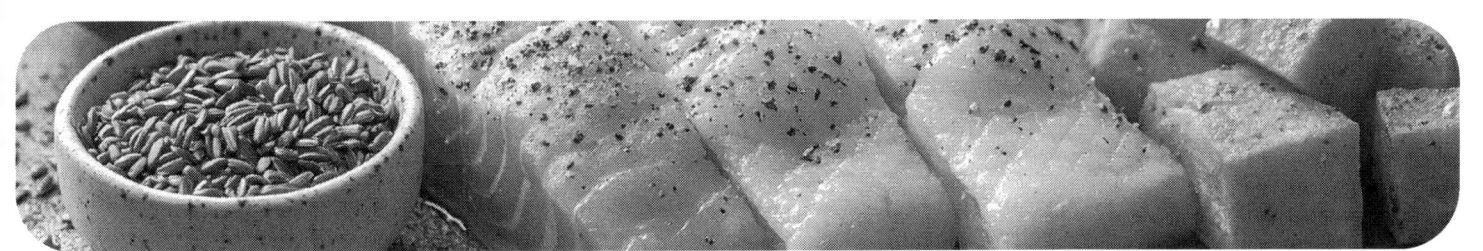

Table of Contents

Introduction

If you're holding this book, chances are you're tired—tired of the discomfort that creeps in after every meal, tired of guessing which foods might cause that familiar burning in your chest, and tired of navigating the maze of conflicting advice about acid reflux and diet. Whether you've been diagnosed with GERD (gastroesophageal reflux disease) or are managing chronic acid reflux symptoms on your own, you're not alone—and you're not without hope.

As a nutritionist and cookbook author who has worked closely with individuals dealing with digestive disorders, I understand how overwhelming and frustrating this journey can be. Acid reflux isn't just a minor inconvenience. It can disrupt your meals, your sleep, and your overall quality of life. You may have found yourself staring at a plate of food, wondering, «Will this hurt me later?» — or giving up on cooking altogether because it feels too complicated, too uncertain, or too exhausting.

That's precisely why I created The Acid Reflux Diet Cookbook for Beginners. This book is your gentle guide to reclaiming your meals, your comfort, and your confidence—one soothing, satisfying recipe at a time. Here, you'll find straightforward and reliable recipes crafted with intention. Each dish is carefully crafted to be gentle on your digestive system, free from common reflux triggers such as citrus, tomatoes, spicy seasonings, and heavy fats. But don't worry — you won't have to sacrifice flavor or nourishment.

You don't need to be an experienced cook to benefit from this cookbook. I've kept every recipe beginner-friendly, using familiar and accessible ingredients and simple techniques that fit easily into busy lifestyles. Whether you're preparing a weekday dinner, a quick breakfast, or a cozy weekend meal, you'll have the tools you need to cook with clarity and care. No guesswork. No stress. Just meals that help you feel better—physically and emotionally.

This book isn't just about food; it's about empowerment. It's about knowing that what you eat can support your body rather than working against it. With every meal you make, you're giving yourself the gift of relief, balance, and a sense of control over your health. So take a deep breath. You've already taken the first step by opening this book. Together, we'll make this new way of eating not only manageable but enjoyable. You've got this— and I'm here to help every step of the way.

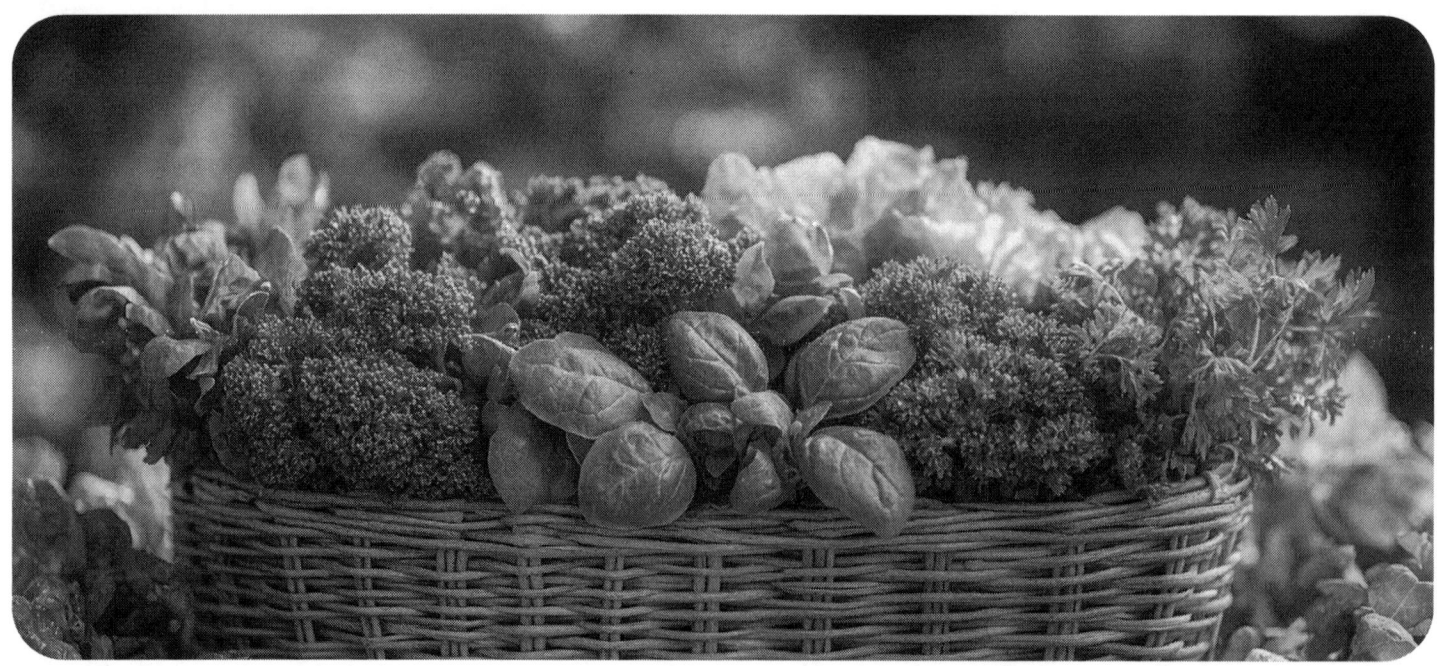

Chapter 1: Understanding and Thriving on the Acid Reflux Diet

If you've ever felt a burning sensation in your chest after eating, or had a sour taste rise in your throat, you've likely experienced **acid reflux**. While occasional reflux is common and not usually cause for concern, **chronic acid reflux** can become disruptive and even harmful over time. When it occurs regularly — more than twice a week — it may be diagnosed as **Gastroesophageal Reflux Disease (GERD)**.

So, what exactly is happening in your body when this occurs?

At the base of your esophagus (the tube that carries food from your mouth to your stomach) is a small ring of muscle called the **lower esophageal sphincter (LES)**. Its job is to open to let food into your stomach and then close tightly to keep stomach acid where it belongs — in your stomach. But sometimes, that muscle weakens or relaxes at the wrong time. When that happens, **acid can backflow** into the esophagus, causing the uncomfortable symptoms commonly referred to as acid reflux.

Common Symptoms of Acid Reflux and GERD

- A burning sensation in the chest (heartburn)
- A sour or bitter taste in the mouth
- Burping or belching after meals
- Regurgitation of food or liquid
- Bloating and stomach discomfort
- Chronic cough or sore throat
- Hoarseness or a feeling of a lump in the throat

These symptoms may worsen after eating large meals, lying down too soon after eating, or consuming trigger foods (which we'll explore in depth soon).

Left unmanaged, chronic reflux can damage the lining of the esophagus and increase the risk of complications like **esophagitis, Barrett's esophagus,** or even **esophageal cancer** in rare cases. But here's the good news: **diet and lifestyle changes can have a powerful impact** — often enough to reduce or eliminate symptoms without medication.

Why Food Choices Matter

Every meal you eat has the potential to cither **support or irritate your digestive health.** Certain foods are known to relax the LES or stimulate excess stomach acid. Others create gas and pressure that push acid up. Even healthy foods — such as citrus, tomatoes, or garlic — can be problematic for individuals with reflux. So managing acid reflux isn't about "eating clean" in a general sense — it's about learning which specific foods are gentle on your digestive system and which are not.

Food isn't the only factor, but for many people, **it's the most manageable and most impactful.** And unlike medications, food choices come with side benefits — such as improved energy, a healthier weight, better sleep, and reduced overall health risks.

The Goal of the Acid Reflux Diet

At its core, the acid reflux diet is designed to help your body **heal and stay balanced.** It aims to:

- **Avoid trigger foods** that aggravate the esophagus or increase acid production.
- **Support digestion** by choosing gentle, nourishing ingredients.
- **Encourage smaller, balanced meals** throughout the day.
- **Reduce inflammation** and irritation in the digestive tract.

This diet is not a fad, and it's not about restriction for the sake of weight loss. It's a

functional, healing approach to eating. The idea is to **calm your digestive system**, give your body what it needs to heal, and help you feel better after every meal — not worse.

Beyond Spicy Food: Unexpected Triggers

Most people think of spicy food when they hear "acid reflux," but that's just the beginning. You might be surprised to learn that **many common and even nutritious ingredients** can cause issues.

Examples include:

- **Tomatoes and tomato-based products** – naturally acidic and often a top trigger
- **Citrus fruits** – oranges, lemons, grapefruits, and their juices
- **Chocolate** – contains both caffeine and a compound called theobromine, which can relax the LES
- **Garlic and onions** – especially raw- can irritate the esophagus
- **Caffeine and carbonated drinks** – they increase pressure in the stomach and LES relaxation
- **Peppermint and spearmint** – often found in teas and candies, they seem soothing but actually worsen reflux

These foods aren't "bad" in general — they're just **not right for reflux-sensitive individuals.** And while it may feel discouraging at first to limit familiar favorites, there are **plenty of flavorful, satisfying alternatives** that won't leave you feeling deprived.

Why This Cookbook Works

This cookbook is designed to make this way of eating simple, flexible, and **enjoyable**. You won't find confusing restrictions or unrealistic meal plans here. Instead, you'll get:

- **Clear guidance** on what to eat and what to avoid
- **Reflux-friendly recipe options** for breakfast, lunch, dinner, snacks, and even desserts
- **Practical cooking tips** for reducing acidity and supporting digestion
- **Ingredient swaps** that allow you to recreate favorites without the flare-ups
- **Meal planning support** to help you stay consistent without stress

Every recipe in this book was created with digestive comfort in mind — using real, everyday ingredients that are easy to find and simple to prepare.

Listening to Your Body

The truth is, **every person is a little different.** Some people can tolerate small amounts of certain trigger foods; others can't. That's why a one-size-fits-all approach doesn't work.

As you begin this journey, it's helpful to:

- **Keep a food and symptom journal**
- **Track patterns** between what you eat and how you feel
- **Adjust your meals** based on your personal needs

You may discover that small changes — such as eating dinner earlier, swapping tomato sauce for red pepper purée, or switching to herbal tea — can make a **significant difference** in how you feel.

The Takeaway

Acid reflux and GERD can disrupt your quality of life — but they don't have to control it. With the right information and tools, you can **manage your symptoms naturally** and still enjoy delicious, satisfying meals. The acid reflux diet isn't about giving things up — it's about gaining back your comfort, your energy, and your peace of mind.

By understanding what reflux is, how food plays a role, and what your body needs to feel its best, you're already on the path toward healing.

Identifying Your Triggers: Foods to Avoid and Why

One of the most important steps in managing acid reflux through diet is learning which foods trigger your symptoms. While the acid reflux diet offers general guidelines, **your personal triggers may vary.** That's why identifying what causes your flare-ups is key to reducing discomfort and healing your digestive system.

Let's start by looking at **why certain foods cause problems.**

When you eat, your body produces stomach acid to help break down food. In people with reflux, this acid can escape upward into the esophagus — especially if **the lower esophageal sphincter (LES),** a ring-like muscle that separates the esophagus from the stomach, becomes relaxed or weakened.

Some foods contribute to this process by:
- Relaxing the LES
- Increasing stomach acid production
- Causing the stomach to expand or bloat (putting pressure on the LES)
- Irritating the lining of the esophagus

These effects can happen even when the food is considered "healthy." So while it might seem counterintuitive, a spinach salad with citrus vinaigrette and garlic croutons might trigger reflux in someone sensitive, even though every ingredient is nutrient-rich.

Common Trigger Foods and Why They Matter

Here's a practical breakdown of foods that are commonly linked to acid reflux, along with why they tend to cause trouble.

1. Fried and Fatty Foods

Examples: French fries, fried chicken, bacon, sausage, buttery pastries

Why: High-fat foods slow digestion, increase acid production, and relax the LES.

2. Spicy Foods

Examples: Chili peppers, hot sauce, cayenne, curry, wasabi

Why: Spices can irritate the esophageal lining and stimulate acid release.

3. Citrus Fruits and Juices

Examples: Oranges, lemons, limes, grapefruits, pineapple

Why: These fruits are naturally high in acid, which can irritate the esophagus and worsen heartburn.

4. Tomatoes and Tomato-Based Products

Examples: Pasta sauce, salsa, ketchup, tomato soup

Why: Tomatoes are acidic and commonly cause flare-ups, especially when cooked or concentrated.

5. Chocolate

Why: Chocolate contains caffeine, fat, and a compound called theobromine — all of which can relax the LES and stimulate acid.

6. Caffeine

Examples: Coffee, black tea, energy drinks

Why: Caffeine increases stomach acid and can weaken the LES. Even decaf coffee may be irritating due to its acidity.

7. **Carbonated Beverages**

Examples: Soda, sparkling water, fizzy juices

Why: Bubbles expand in the stomach, increasing pressure and pushing acid upward.

8. **Garlic and Onions**

Why: These flavorful staples are common triggers for many people, especially when raw. They may irritate the esophagus and promote gas.

9. **Peppermint and Mint-Flavored Products**

Examples: Peppermint tea, mints, mint gum

Why: Though often used for soothing digestion, mint can relax the LES and allow acid to rise.

10. **Alcohol**

Examples: Wine, beer, cocktails, hard liquor

Why: Alcohol can relax the LES, irritate the esophagus, and increase acid production.

The Power of Personalization

Although this list provides a starting point, **not everyone reacts in the same way**. You might tolerate a small amount of tomato or onion, while someone else experiences a flare-up from just a few bites. That's why one of the most valuable tools in this journey is a **food-symptom diary.**

How to Keep a Food and Symptom Diary

Start simple. Here's how it works:

- **Write down everything you eat and drink** each day — meals, snacks, drinks, condiments, sauces.
- **Record the time of day** you ate each item.
- **Note any symptoms** (heartburn, bloating, coughing, throat irritation) and the time they occurred.
- **Look for patterns.** Did symptoms follow a particular food within an hour or two? Did eating late make things worse?

Use this journal to highlight both your triggers and your safe foods. You'll be surprised how much clarity this simple practice can bring.

Watch for Combination Effects

Sometimes, a food might not bother you on its own, but it becomes a problem when combined with other substances. For example:

- A tomato slice on a sandwich might be okay — but with garlic mayo and a carbonated drink? Trouble.
- A cup of herbal tea may be fine — unless it's peppermint.

Paying attention to how different ingredients interact can help you make smart choices and prevent surprise flare-ups.

"Healthy" Doesn't Always Mean Reflux-Safe

One of the most frustrating parts of managing acid reflux is realizing that some nutritious foods can still make you feel terrible. For example:

- **Avocado** – full of healthy fats, but those fats can relax the LES
- **Citrus fruits** – rich in vitamin C, but acidic
- **Garlic and onions** – packed with antioxidants, but irritating for many

That's why it's essential to shift your mindset. You're not giving up on health — **you're**

redefining health to include how your body feels after eating.

What to Do If You Have Multiple Triggers

It can feel overwhelming if you react to many of the foods you used to enjoy. Here are a few ways to manage that:

- **Start with an elimination phase.** Remove common triggers for 2–3 weeks, then reintroduce one at a time to test your tolerance.
- **Focus on what you can eat.** Many gentle, nourishing options won't trigger symptoms.
- **Keep your meals simple** — fewer ingredients make it easier to identify triggers.

You're in Control

Discovering your food triggers puts the power in your hands. Instead of guessing or reacting after the fact, you'll begin to **anticipate what your body needs** and respond with confidence.

Consider this a learning process. It takes time, patience, and self-awareness, but you'll gain something invaluable: a sense of control over your health.

Building Your Pantry: Safe Ingredients and Smart Swaps

Creating a reflux-friendly kitchen is one of the most crucial steps in effectively managing your symptoms. When your pantry and fridge are stocked with supportive ingredients, making safe, healing meals becomes second nature — even on your busiest days.

This section will walk you through what to keep on hand, how to make smart substitutions, and how to shop and cook with confidence. It's not about perfection — it's about being prepared.

Stocking the Reflux-Friendly Kitchen

When it comes to acid reflux, simplicity and balance are your best allies. Choose whole, minimally processed foods, and steer clear of high-fat, high-acid, and spicy items. Here's what to keep around:

Pantry Staples:
- Old-fashioned oats or steel-cut oatmeal
- Brown rice, quinoa, couscous, bulgur
- Whole wheat or gluten-free pasta (no added tomato powder)
- Unsalted rice cakes, whole grain crackers
- Canned beans (rinsed), lentils
- Mild broths: vegetable or low-sodium chicken

Fruits (low-acid):
- Bananas
- Apples (peeled)
- Melons: cantaloupe, honeydew, watermelon
- Pears
- Non-citrus dried fruits: apricots, dates (in moderation)

Vegetables (gentle and low-acid):
- Zucchini, carrots, green beans
- Sweet potatoes, pumpkin,

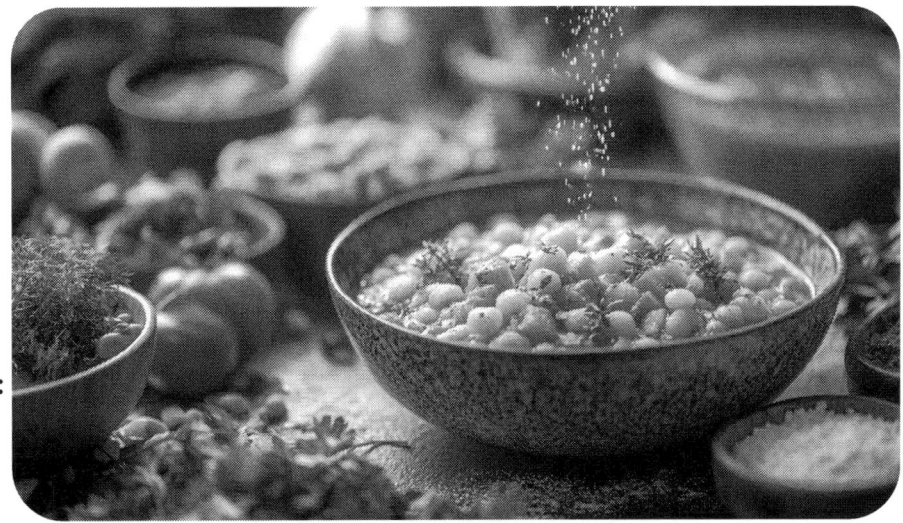

squash
- Cabbage (cooked), broccoli (in small amounts)
- Leafy greens: romaine, spinach, arugula (not mustard greens)

Proteins:
- Skinless chicken or turkey breast
- White fish: cod, tilapia, haddock
- Eggs (especially egg whites)
- Tofu, tempeh
- Low-fat cottage cheese or yogurt

Dairy/Alternatives:
- Almond milk, oat milk, rice milk (unsweetened)
- Low-fat or lactose-free dairy options

Herbs and Spices (non-irritating):
- Basil, parsley, oregano, thyme, rosemary
- Ginger and turmeric (small amounts)
- Fennel, cinnamon (used sparingly)

Smart Ingredient Swaps

Even minor substitutions can reduce irritation and improve digestion. Here are some reflux-friendly swaps to keep in mind:
- **Lemon juice** → apple cider vinegar (diluted, used sparingly)
- **Tomato sauce** → roasted red pepper purée or carrot purée
- **Spicy condiments (sriracha, hot sauce)** → mashed avocado with herbs
- **Mayonnaise or sour cream** → plain low-fat Greek yogurt
- **Garlic or onion** → chive tops or asafoetida (in tiny amounts)
- **Coffee** → herbal teas: chamomile, ginger, fennel

Tips for Shopping Smart

Reading labels becomes second nature once you know what to avoid. Here's what to watch for:
- **Avoid added acids:** citric acid, vinegar, lemon juice, "sour" flavors
- **Watch for spices:** many packaged foods list "spices" without specifying — these may include black pepper or chili
- **Check for added fat or oils:** especially in pre-made dressings, sauces, or snacks
- **Go low-sodium when possible:** salt isn't a reflux trigger, but high sodium can contribute to bloating

Batch Cooking and Freezer Prep

When your pantry and fridge are well stocked, you can batch cook base ingredients like:
- Brown rice or quinoa
- Roasted or steamed vegetables
- Baked chicken breast
- Soups or purees (carrot-ginger, zucchini-basil)

Divide into single portions and freeze. Having go-to meals on hand makes reflux-safe eating easier on busy or low-energy days.

Flavor Without the Burn

You don't need heavy spices or acids to make food delicious. Try layering flavors with:
Roasted vegetables (natural sweetness)

Fresh herbs

Low-acid ingredients like cucumber, fennel, or cooked leeks

Healthy fats like avocado (in moderation) or olive oil

Bonus Tip: Use vegetable or bone broth as a base for flavor instead of heavy sauces. Simmer with ginger, parsley, or celery for depth without irritation.

A well-stocked kitchen is your first line of defense against flare-ups. When everything you need is already on hand, cooking becomes less stressful and more intuitive. By using smart swaps, gentle seasonings, and reflux-friendly staples, you can turn your kitchen into a space for healing and nourishment.

Cooking Methods That Support Digestion

When it comes to managing acid reflux, **what you cook is important — but how you cook it can be just as critical.** You might select all the right reflux-safe ingredients, but if they're fried in heavy oil, charred on the grill, or heavily seasoned with irritants, the result could still trigger symptoms.

This section will guide you through reflux-friendly cooking techniques that support digestion, reduce acid production, and help soothe your system — all while maintaining flavor, texture, and variety.

Why Cooking Methods Matter

Cooking changes the structure of food. It affects how easily food is digested, how acidic it becomes during digestion, and whether it will relax the lower esophageal sphincter (LES) - the small muscle that keeps stomach acid in its place.

Certain cooking methods — like frying or blackening — can:

- Increase fat content (which delays digestion and increases pressure on the LES)
- Produce compounds that irritate the esophagus
- Remove water content, making foods harder to digest
- Intensify spices and acidity

In contrast, **gentle cooking methods** preserve the food's moisture, reduce irritation, and promote better digestion — all essential for managing acid reflux and GERD.

Best Cooking Methods for Acid Reflux

1. Steaming

Steaming uses hot vapor to cook food while preserving moisture and nutrients.

Best for: vegetables, white fish, skinless poultry, soft grains

Benefits:

- No added fat required
- Keeps food moist and easy to swallow
- Reduces the risk of overcooking or burning

Pro tip: Add herbs like parsley or dill to the steaming water to lightly infuse flavor without irritation.

2. Baking (at moderate temperature)

Baking is great for evenly cooking proteins, vegetables, and whole grains without added oil.

Best for: chicken breasts, roasted vegetables, casseroles, baked oatmeal

Benefits:
- Requires little or no fat
- Keeps ingredients separate (great for meal prep)
- Allows for gentle, slow cooking that prevents charring

Tip: Avoid broiling or baking at very high temperatures, which can dry out food and create acidic, burnt edges.

3. Poaching

Poaching is the process of gently simmering food in water or broth.

Best for: eggs, poultry, fish, apples or pears (for desserts)

Benefits:
- Keeps food very soft and moist
- Easy to digest
- No added oil required

Lifehack: Poach fruits like pears or apples with cinnamon and a splash of vanilla for a reflux-safe dessert.

4. Slow Cooking

Slow cookers (or crockpots) are one of the most useful tools in a reflux-friendly kitchen.

Best for: stews, soups, oatmeal, beans, shredded chicken

Benefits:
- Breaks down fibers for easier digestion
- Uses minimal fat and gentle heat
- Reduces hands-on time — great for busy schedules

Essential tip: Avoid adding acidic ingredients (like tomatoes or vinegar) to slow cooker recipes. Use veggie stock, root vegetables, and reflux-safe herbs instead.

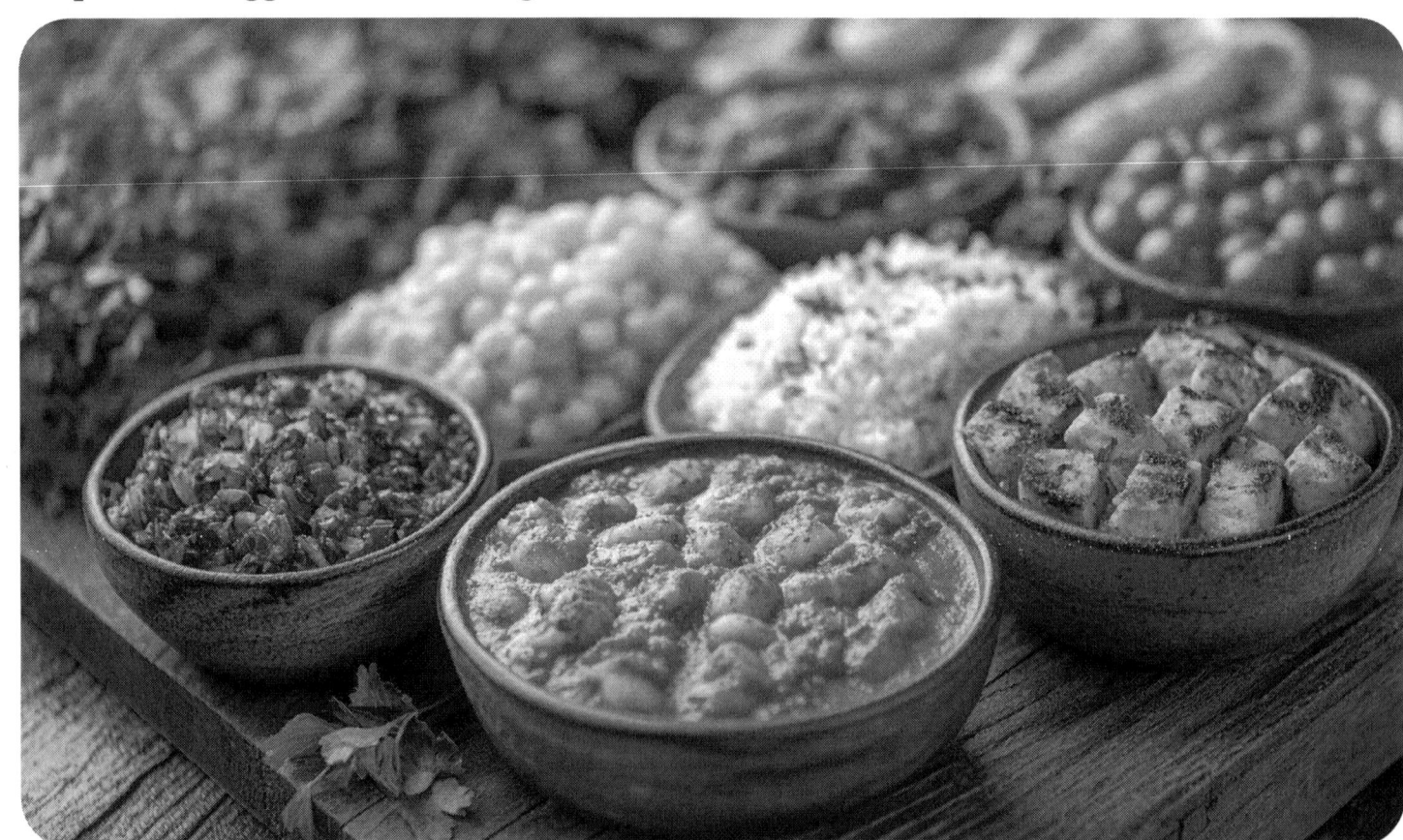

5. Light Grilling or Roasting (without charring)

Grilling can work if done carefully — avoid high flames and charring.

Best for: poultry, zucchini, bell peppers, peaches

Tips:
- Use foil or grill trays to avoid drippings and smoke
- Marinate with reflux-safe options (like olive oil and herbs — no citrus or garlic)
- Flip often to prevent blackened edges

Methods to Avoid or Use Cautiously

1) Deep-Frying

Why it's a problem:
- Adds a large amount of fat
- Fat slows digestion and increases acid production
- Food becomes heavy and greasy, which can relax the LES

Examples: fried chicken, French fries, doughnuts

2) Pan-Frying in Butter or Oil

Even healthy oils like olive oil can be problematic if used excessively or heated too high.

Why it's a problem:
- High heat can degrade oils, creating compounds that irritate the stomach and esophagus
- Adds unnecessary fat

Alternative: use nonstick cookware and low-sodium vegetable broth to sauté or "steam-fry."

3) Blackening, Charring, or Searing

These techniques often involve very high heat and lead to burnt edges or crispy exteriors.

Why it's a problem:
- Charred foods may contain compounds that irritate the GI tract
- The texture is harder to digest
- Often associated with over-seasoning and high-fat marinades

Flavor Without the Flare-Ups

Many people worry that gentle cooking means bland food. That's not true. You can still enjoy vibrant, satisfying meals — the key is to build flavor in reflux-safe ways.

Use these instead of spicy or acidic ingredients:
- Fresh herbs: parsley, basil, thyme, oregano, dill
- Mild spices: turmeric, ginger, cinnamon (use cautiously), coriander
- Aromatics: green onion tops (not the bulb), leeks (lightly cooked), fennel
- Flavor bases: low-sodium veggie or bone broth, carrot purée, roasted red pepper purée

Bonus tip: A splash of rice vinegar or apple cider vinegar (diluted and used in tiny amounts) can offer brightness without triggering reflux — for some people. Test cautiously.

Healthy Habits Around Cooking and Eating

Cooking methods matter — but so do your habits around meals. Here are key practices to support digestion and reduce reflux risk:

1. Eat slowly and chew thoroughly: Digestion begins in the mouth. The more you chew,

the easier your stomach can process food.

2. **Cook in smaller batches:** Reheat only what you need. Reheated meals can become dry and harder to digest.
3. **Avoid eating right before bed:** Wait 2–3 hours after eating before lying down. This gives your stomach time to empty.
4. **Portion control matters:** Overeating increases pressure on the LES. Use smaller plates to help manage portions.
5. **Stay upright after meals:** Sit, walk gently, or stretch — avoid reclining.

Appliances That Can Help

Investing in a few reflux-friendly tools can make cooking easier and more effective:

- **Slow cooker:** Great for hands-free, gentle meals
- **Steamer basket or electric steamer:** Easy, quick cooking with no added fat
- **Nonstick cookware:** Reduces need for oil
- **Blender or food processor:** Helps create smooth, easy-to-digest sauces, soups, and purées

Reflux-Safe Meal Examples by Cooking Method

Steamed:

- Steamed zucchini and carrots with grilled turkey breast
- Steamed white fish with soft rice and herbs

Baked:

- Baked oatmeal with mashed banana and cinnamon
- Chicken and rice casserole with steamed greens

Slow Cooked:

- Turkey and vegetable stew with barley
- Creamy carrot and sweet potato soup

Poached:

- Poached egg on toast with mashed avocado (if tolerated)
- Poached pear with warm almond milk and oats

Conclusion: Gentle Cooking, Powerful Results

Learning how to cook for acid reflux isn't about sacrificing taste or convenience — it's about **making smart choices that soothe your body and support long-term health.** By shifting toward gentle, low-fat, moist cooking techniques and adjusting your kitchen habits, you can enjoy meals that satisfy without causing pain.

You don't need fancy tools or chef skills. You need simple methods, a bit of planning, and a mindset focused on healing — one recipe at a time.

Making It Work: Routines, Meal Planning & Eating Out

Adopting a new way of eating — especially for health reasons — can feel overwhelming at first. You may wonder: *How will I stick to this when life gets busy? What if my family eats differently? How do I eat out or travel without risking a flare-up?*

The good news is: **it doesn't have to be complicated.** With a bit of planning and a few simple routines, the acid reflux diet can become a natural part of your day — not a stressful chore. This section gives you practical tools to make it all manageable, flexible, and sustainable, even if you're short on time or cooking confidence.

Why Consistency Matters

The acid reflux diet isn't a short-term fix — it's a lifestyle that supports long-term digestive healing and symptom control. But it only works if you stick with it consistently.

Consistency doesn't mean perfection. It means doing your best most of the time — and being prepared, so you're not caught off guard when hunger strikes or your schedule gets hectic.

That's where routines come in.

Simple Daily Habits That Support Digestive Health

Start with a few manageable changes that build a foundation for long-term success:

- **Eat smaller, more frequent meals** – Instead of 2 or 3 large meals, aim for 4–5 light meals throughout the day. This eases pressure on the stomach and LES.
- **Avoid eating late at night** – Finish your last meal or snack at least **2–3 hours before going to bed**. This helps prevent nighttime reflux.
- **Sit upright after eating** – Stay seated or lightly active for 30–60 minutes after meals.
- **Chew food thoroughly and eat slowly** – Digestion begins in the mouth. Slow eating reduces the chance of overeating and bloating.
- **Drink fluids between meals, not during** – Too much liquid with meals can expand the stomach and increase pressure.

These small habits make a big difference — and they're easy to build into your day once you become more aware of them.

Meal Planning for Busy People

Planning your meals may sound like a lot of work, but it actually saves you time, stress, and energy — especially when you're adjusting to a new way of eating.

Here's how to make it easy and realistic:

Step 1: Choose 3–5 core meals per week

You don't need to plan every bite — just identify a few reliable meals you enjoy and rotate them. Include options for breakfast, lunch, and dinner.

Example:
- Oatmeal with banana and almond milk (breakfast)
- Rice bowl with turkey, zucchini, and carrots (lunch or dinner)
- Baked sweet potatoes with steamed greens and white fish (dinner)

Step 2: Make a shopping list

Shop for the week based on your chosen meals. Stock up on pantry staples, such as rice, oats, frozen vegetables, and lean proteins. This ensures you're never far from a reflux-safe meal.

Step 3: Prep ingredients ahead
- Chop vegetables and store them in containers
- Cook grains like rice or quinoa in bulk
- Roast or steam proteins and portion them for grab-and-go meals
- Make and freeze soups or stews in single servings

Tip: Set aside 1–2 hours each week (e.g., Sunday afternoon) for prep. Put on music or a podcast — it can become a relaxing routine!

Eating Out Without the Worry

Dining out can be tricky when you're managing acid reflux, but it doesn't have to be off-limits. With a little strategy and confidence, you can still enjoy meals out with family and friends.

Before You Go
- **Check the menu online** – Look for baked, grilled, or steamed options.
- **Call ahead if needed** – Ask about ingredients or possible substitutions.

At the Restaurant
- **Request sauce or dressing on the side** – Many sauces are acidic or spicy. Ask for olive oil and herbs instead.
- **Choose grilled or baked proteins** – Avoid fried or breaded dishes.
- **Skip spicy condiments, citrus marinades, and raw onions.**
- **Opt for plain sides,** such as rice, steamed vegetables, or baked potatoes.
- **Watch portion sizes** – Ask for a to-go box upfront and portion out your meal.

Words to look for on the menu:
- "Steamed," "roasted," "grilled" (no char)
- "Plain," "light," "oil-free"
- Avoid terms like "crispy," "zesty," "blackened," "spicy," "buffalo," or "sautéed in butter."

Managing Family Meals When Not Everyone Eats the Same

If you live with others who don't follow the acid reflux diet, it can feel tricky to prepare meals that work for everyone. The solution? **Build meals around reflux-safe bases** — then let others customize.

Example: Build-Your-Own Bowl Night
- Base: rice or couscous
- Protein: grilled chicken or tofu
- Toppings: cooked vegetables, plain yogurt sauce
- Optional extras (for others): spicy sauces, cheese, tomatoes, etc.

This approach keeps your meal safe — and everyone else satisfied.

Tip: Label your meal containers or prep portions separately if needed. Batch cooking makes this much easier.

Freezer Meals and Emergency Options

Some days, you just don't feel like cooking — and that's okay. That's why having **emergency reflux-friendly meals** in the freezer can save the day.

Great freezer options:
- Chicken and rice soup
- Turkey and sweet potato stew
- Baked oatmeal cups with pears or apples
- Cooked brown rice and steamed veggies in single-serve containers

Also, keep **snacks on hand:**
- Rice cakes
- Bananas or peeled apples
- Plain oatmeal packets
- Boiled eggs

- Low-fat yogurt

Pro tip: Freeze in small, meal-sized containers so you can defrost just what you need at a time.

Tracking Progress and Staying Motivated

As you build new routines, it's helpful to track your meals and symptoms. This isn't about perfection — it's about learning what works for your body.

Use a simple notebook or app to:
- Log what you eat
- Record when and how symptoms appear
- Note how certain meals make you feel

Over time, you'll build a personal reflux-friendly eating strategy that works just for you.

Celebrate small wins — like a day without heartburn, a new recipe you enjoy, or a successful restaurant outing. Progress builds momentum.

Conclusion: Your Lifestyle, Your Control

Staying consistent with the acid reflux diet isn't about rigid rules or stress — it's about building small, steady habits that work in your real life.

With a little planning, prep, and flexibility, you'll find that **eating for reflux relief becomes second nature.** You don't have to cook elaborate meals or completely overhaul your life. You simply need to establish routines that support your well-being.

This journey is about more than avoiding discomfort — it's about reclaiming your energy, your confidence, and your joy in food.

You've got this. And I'm here to guide you every step of the way.

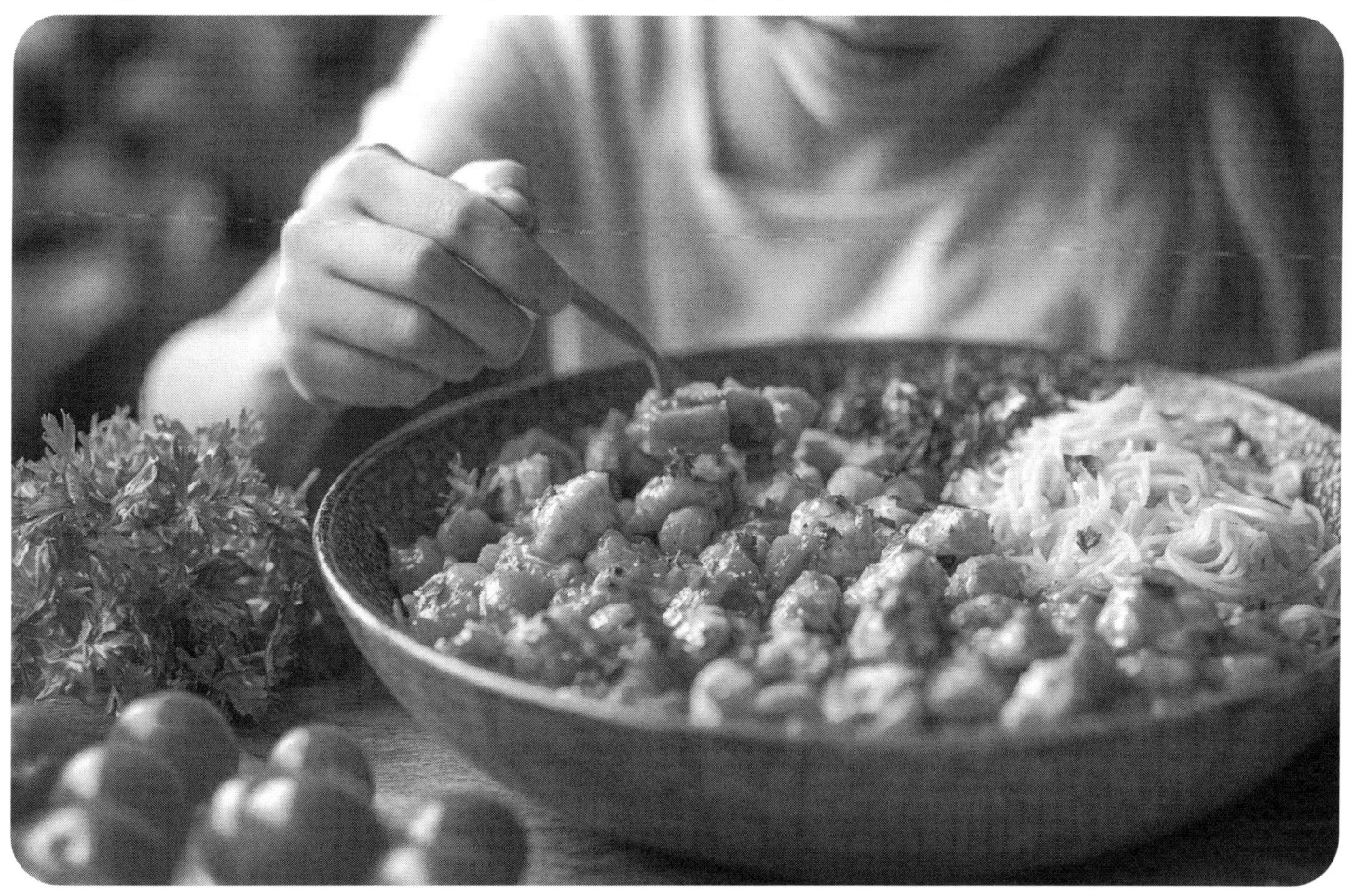

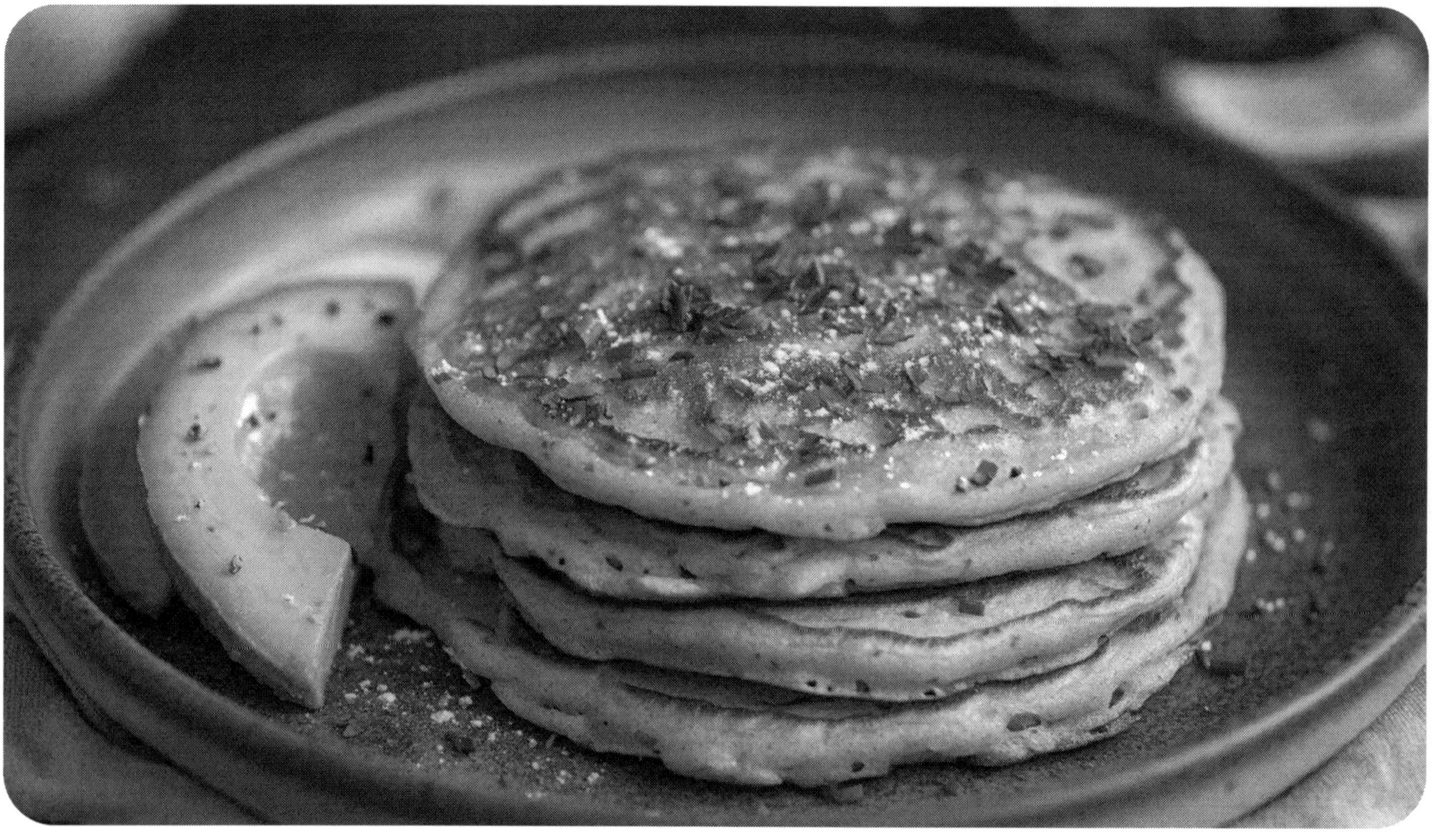

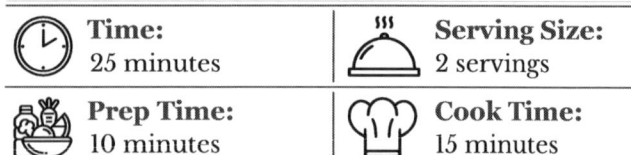

Chapter 2: Breakfast

Chickpea Flour Pancakes with Fresh Herbs

	Time: 25 minutes		Serving Size: 2 servings
	Prep Time: 10 minutes		Cook Time: 15 minutes

Each Serving Has:
Calories: 192, Carbohydrates: 23g, Saturated Fat: 0.5g, Protein: 9g, Fat: 7g, Sodium: 213mg, Potassium: 313mg, Fiber: 4g, Sugar: 3g, Vitamin C: 9mg, Calcium: 24mg, Iron: 2mg

Ingredients:
- 1/2 cup [60g] sifted chickpea flour
- 1/2 cup [120ml] water
- 2 tbsp chopped fresh parsley
- 1 tbsp chopped fresh dill
- 1/4 cup [25g] grated zucchini, squeezed dry
- 2 tbsp grated carrot
- 1 tbsp chopped cooked leek, cooled
- 1/4 tsp ground turmeric
- 1 tsp olive oil

Directions:
1. In a medium mixing bowl, whisk together sifted chickpea flour, water, and ground turmeric until smooth and lump-free.
2. Fold in chopped parsley, dill, cooked leek, grated zucchini, and carrot until evenly combined.
3. Heat 1 teaspoon of olive oil in a non-stick skillet over medium heat.
4. Pour half the batter into the skillet, gently spreading it into a round pancake about 6 inches [15 cm] in diameter. Cook for 3–4 minutes, or until the edges appear dry and the bottom is lightly golden.
5. Flip the pancake carefully using a spatula and cook for an additional 3–4 minutes, until the center is set and golden brown on both sides.
6. Repeat with the remaining batter to make the second pancake. Serve warm.

Amaranth Porridge with Vanilla and Blueberries

Time: 30 minutes	Serving Size: 2 servings
Prep Time: 5 minutes	Cook Time: 25 minutes

Each Serving Has:

Calories: 236, Carbohydrates: 39g, Saturated Fat: 0.3g, Protein: 7g, Fat: 6g, Sodium: 86mg, Potassium: 274mg, Fiber: 5g, Sugar: 7g, Vitamin C: 4mg, Calcium: 100mg, Iron: 3mg

Ingredients:

- 1/2 cup [95g] rinsed amaranth
- 1 1/2 cups [360ml] unsweetened oat milk
- 1/2 tsp vanilla extract
- 1/2 cup [75g]
- mixed fresh blueberries
- 1 tbsp maple syrup
- 1 tbsp ground flaxseed
- 1/4 tsp ground cinnamon

Directions:

1. In a medium saucepan, combine rinsed amaranth and oat milk.
2. Bring the mixture to a gentle boil over medium heat, then reduce to low and cover.
3. Simmer for 20–25 minutes, stirring occasionally, until the amaranth is tender and the mixture has thickened to a creamy consistency.
4. Stir in vanilla extract, fresh blueberries, maple syrup, ground flaxseed, and ground cinnamon until well incorporated.
5. Cook for an additional 2 minutes over low heat, stirring gently to warm the blueberries without breaking them down completely.
6. Divide the porridge evenly between two bowls and serve warm.

Sweet Potato and Spinach Breakfast Bowl

Time: 25 minutes	Serving Size: 2 bowls
Prep Time: 10 minutes	Cook Time: 15 minutes

Each Serving Has:

Calories: 280, Carbohydrates: 45g, Saturated Fat: 1g, Protein: 7g, Fat: 6g, Sodium: 180mg, Potassium: 600mg, Fiber: 8g, Sugar: 10g, Vitamin C: 25mg, Calcium: 50mg, Iron: 2mg.

Ingredients:

- 1 medium sweet potato, peeled and cubed (about 1 cup [200g])
- 1/2 tbsp of olive oil
- 1/4 tsp of ground cinnamon
- 1/8 tsp of ground nutmeg
- 2 cups [60g] of
- fresh spinach
- 1/4 cup [60ml] of unsweetened almond milk
- 1/2 tsp of pure maple syrup
- 2 tbsp of cooked quinoa
- 1 tbsp of unsalted pumpkin seeds

Directions:

1. Preheat your oven to 375°F. Line a baking sheet with parchment paper.
2. Toss sweet potato cubes with olive oil, cinnamon, and nutmeg in a bowl. Spread in a single layer on a baking sheet. Roast for 15 minutes, flipping halfway, until tender and caramelized.
3. While the sweet potatoes roast, place spinach in a skillet over medium heat. Add 2 tablespoons of water and cook for 2-3 minutes, stirring occasionally, until wilted. Remove from heat and set aside.
4. Heat almond milk in a saucepan over low heat until warm. Stir in maple syrup and set aside.
5. Once the sweet potatoes are cooked, assemble the bowls. Add wilted spinach, cooked quinoa, and warm almond milk mixture.
6. Top with a sprinkle of pumpkin seeds.

Rice Porridge with Banana and Cinnamon

 Time:
20 minutes

 Serving Size:
2 bowls

 Prep Time:
5 minutes

 Cook Time:
15 minutes

Each Serving Has:

Calories: 230, Carbohydrates: 48g, Saturated Fat: 0.5g, Protein: 4g, Fat: 2g, Sodium: 50mg, Potassium: 400mg, Fiber: 3g, Sugar: 12g, Vitamin C: 5mg, Calcium: 60mg, Iron: 1mg.

Ingredients:

- 1/2 cup [100g] of cooked white rice (preferably short-grain or jasmine)
- 1 cup [240ml] of unsweetened almond milk
- 1/2 tsp of pure vanilla extract
- 1/4 tsp of ground cinnamon
- 1 tbsp of pure maple syrup
- 1 medium ripe banana, sliced
- 1/2 tbsp of unsweetened shredded coconut (for garnish)
- 1/4 tsp of ground flaxseed (optional)

Directions:

1. In a saucepan, combine cooked white rice and almond milk. Heat over medium, stirring gently to combine.
2. Add vanilla extract, cinnamon, and maple syrup to the mixture. Stir well and bring to a gentle simmer.
3. Reduce heat to low and cook for 10-12 minutes, stirring occasionally, until the porridge thickens to your desired consistency
4. While the porridge cooks, slice the banana into thin rounds and set aside. Toast shredded coconut in a dry skillet over medium heat for 2-3 minutes, stirring frequently, until golden.
5. Once the porridge has thickened, remove it from the heat.
6. Top with banana, toasted shredded coconut, and a dash of ground flaxseed (if using).

Barley and Apple Breakfast Cereal

 Time:
25 minutes

 Serving Size:
2 bowls

 Prep Time:
5 minutes

 Cook Time:
20 minutes

Each Serving Has:

Calories: 260, Carbohydrates: 52g, Saturated Fat: 0.5g, Protein: 6g, Fat: 3g, Sodium: 30mg, Potassium: 350mg, Fiber: 7g, Sugar: 12g, Vitamin C: 8mg, Calcium: 40mg, Iron: 2mg.

Ingredients:

- 1/2 cup [90g] of pearl barley, rinsed
- 1 1/2 cups [360ml] of water
- 1 medium apple, peeled, cored, and diced
- 1/4 tsp of ground cinnamon
- 1/8 tsp of ground nutmeg
- 1 tbsp of pure
- maple syrup
- 1/2 cup [120ml] of unsweetened almond milk
- 1 tbsp of unsalted sunflower seeds (for garnish)
- 1/2 tbsp of unsweetened dried cranberries or raisins (for garnish)

Directions:

1. In a saucepan, combine the rinsed pearl barley and water. Bring to a boil over medium-high heat, then reduce to low, cover, and simmer for 15 minutes, stirring occasionally.
2. While the barley cooks, peel, core, and dice the apple. Add it to the saucepan with the barley during the last 5 minutes of cooking.
3. Stir in cinnamon, nutmeg, and maple syrup. Simmer gently until the barley is tender and the water is fully absorbed.
4. Once the barley and apple mixture is ready, remove from heat and stir in almond milk to create a creamy consistency.
5. Top with sunflower seeds and a few dried cranberries or raisins, if desired.

Millet and Pumpkin Breakfast Bowl

 Time:
25 minutes

 Serving Size:
2 bowls

 Prep Time:
5 minutes

Cook Time:
20 minutes

Each Serving Has:
Calories: 270, Carbohydrates: 48g, Saturated Fat: 0.5g, Protein: 6g, Fat: 4g, Sodium: 40mg, Potassium: 380mg, Fiber: 6g, Sugar: 8g, Vitamin C: 7mg, Calcium: 50mg, Iron: 2mg.

Ingredients:
- 1/2 cup [100g] of uncooked millet
- 1 cup [240ml] of unsweetened almond milk
- 1/2 cup [120ml] of water
- 1/2 cup [120g] of canned unsweetened pumpkin purée
- 1/4 tsp of ground cinnamon
- 1/8 tsp of ground ginger
- 1 tbsp of pure maple syrup
- 1 tbsp of unsalted pumpkin seeds (for garnish)
- 1/2 tbsp of unsweetened shredded coconut (for garnish)

Directions:
1. Rinse the millet under cold water in a fine mesh strainer to remove debris.
2. In a saucepan, combine millet, almond milk, and water. Bring to a gentle boil over medium-high heat.
3. Reduce heat to low, cover, and simmer the millet for 15 minutes, stirring occasionally to prevent sticking.
4. After 15 minutes, add pumpkin purée, cinnamon, ginger, and maple syrup to the millet. Stir well and cook for an additional 5 minutes to meld the flavors and thicken the mixture.
5. Once the millet is tender and creamy, remove it from the heat.
6. Garnish with pumpkin seeds and a touch of shredded coconut.

Zucchini and Herb Scramble

 Time:
15 minutes

 Serving Size:
2 bowls

 Prep Time:
5 minutes

 Cook Time:
10 minutes

Each Serving Has:
Calories: 180, Carbohydrates: 6g, Saturated Fat: 1g, Protein: 12g, Fat: 12g, Sodium: 90mg, Potassium: 350mg, Fiber: 2g, Sugar: 3g, Vitamin C: 15mg, Calcium: 60mg, Iron: 1.5mg.

Ingredients:
- 1 medium zucchini, grated (about 1 cup [150g])
- 4 large eggs
- 1 tbsp of unsweetened almond milk
- 1/4 tsp of ground turmeric
- 1/4 tsp of dried oregano
- 1/4 tsp of dried thyme
- 1/2 tbsp of olive oil
- 1 tbsp of fresh parsley, chopped (for garnish)

Directions:
1. Grate the zucchini and press it between paper towels to remove excess moisture. Set aside.
2. In a bowl, whisk eggs, almond milk, turmeric, oregano, and thyme until well combined.
3. Heat olive oil in a non-stick skillet over medium heat. Add zucchini and sauté for 2-3 minutes, stirring frequently, until slightly softened.
4. Let it set for 30 seconds, then gently stir and fold with a spatula, ensuring the zucchini is evenly distributed. Cook for 2-3 minutes, stirring occasionally, until the eggs are fully cooked but still soft.
5. Remove the skillet from heat and garnish with fresh parsley.

Cauliflower and Parsley Egg Frittata

 Time:
20 minutes

 Prep Time:
5 minutes

Serving Size:
2 servings

Cook Time:
15 minutes

Each Serving Has:

Calories: 200, Carbohydrates: 5g, Saturated Fat: 1g, Protein: 12g, Fat: 14g, Sodium: 90mg, Potassium: 300mg, Fiber: 2g, Sugar: 2g, Vitamin C: 20mg, Calcium: 50mg, Iron: 1.5mg.

Ingredients:
- 1 cup [100g] of finely chopped cauliflower florets
- 4 large eggs
- 2 tbsp of unsweetened almond milk
- 1/4 tsp of ground turmeric
- 1/4 tsp of dried thyme
- 1/4 cup [10g] of fresh parsley, chopped
- 1 tbsp of olive oil

Directions:

1. Preheat the oven to 375°F. Lightly grease a small oven-safe skillet with 1/2 tbsp of olive oil.
2. Heat the remaining 1/2 tbsp of olive oil in the skillet over medium heat. Add cauliflower florets and sauté for 3-4 minutes, stirring occasionally, until slightly softened.
3. In a bowl, whisk together eggs, almond milk, turmeric, thyme, and half of the chopped parsley until well combined.
4. Pour the egg mixture over the sautéed cauliflower, spreading it evenly. Reduce heat to low and cook for 2 minutes to set the bottom of the frittata.
5. Transfer the skillet to the preheated oven and bake for 8-10 minutes, or until the frittata is puffed and the center is firm.
6. Remove the skillet from the oven and let it cool for 2 minutes.
7. Garnish with the remaining chopped parsley.

Buckwheat and Apple Flatbread

 Time:
35 minutes

 Prep Time:
10 minutes

 Serving Size:
2 servings

 Cook Time:
25 minutes

Each Serving Has:

Calories: 207, Carbohydrates: 38g, Saturated Fat: 0.4g, Protein: 6g, Fat: 5g, Sodium: 112mg, Potassium: 243mg, Fiber: 5g, Sugar: 6g, Vitamin C: 3mg, Calcium: 29mg, Iron: 2mg

Ingredients:
- 1/2 cup [60g] buckwheat flour
- 1/4 cup [60ml] unsweetened almond milk
- 1/4 cup [60ml] water
- 1/2 cup [75g]
- grated peeled apple
- 1 tbsp ground flaxseed
- 1 tbsp maple syrup
- 1/4 tsp ground cinnamon
- 1/2 tsp olive oil

Directions:

1. Preheat the oven to 350°F [175°C]. Line a small baking sheet with parchment paper and lightly grease the surface with olive oil.
2. In a medium mixing bowl, whisk together buckwheat flour, almond milk, water, maple syrup, ground flaxseed, and ground cinnamon until a smooth batter forms.
3. Fold in the grated apple, mixing until evenly distributed throughout the batter.
4. Pour the batter onto the prepared baking sheet and spread it into an even rectangle about 1/4 inch [6mm] thick using a spatula.
5. Bake for 22–25 minutes, or until the surface is dry and edges are lightly golden.
6. Remove from the oven and let cool for 5 minutes before slicing into flatbread portions.
7. Serve warm.

Baked Apple Quinoa Casserole

 Time:
40 minutes

 Prep Time:
10 minutes

Serving Size:
2 servings

Cook Time:
30 minutes

Each Serving Has:
Calories: 260, Carbohydrates: 45g, Saturated Fat: 0.5g, Protein: 7g, Fat: 5g, Sodium: 40mg, Potassium: 400mg, Fiber: 6g, Sugar: 12g, Vitamin C: 6mg, Calcium: 50mg, Iron: 2mg.

Ingredients:
- 1/2 cup [90g] of cooked quinoa
- 1 medium apple, peeled, cored, and diced
- 1/2 cup [120ml] of unsweetened almond milk
- 1/2 tsp of pure vanilla extract
- 1/4 tsp of ground cinnamon
- 1/8 tsp of ground nutmeg
- 1 tbsp of pure maple syrup
- 1 tbsp of unsweetened shredded coconut (for garnish)
- 1 tbsp of chopped unsalted walnuts or almonds (for garnish)

Directions:
1. Preheat your oven to 350°F. Lightly grease a small baking dish with oil or cooking spray.
2. In a mixing bowl, combine quinoa, apple, almond milk, vanilla extract, cinnamon, nutmeg, and maple syrup. Stir until evenly combined.
3. Pour the quinoa and apple mixture into the prepared baking dish, spreading it out into an even layer.
4. Bake the casserole for 25-30 minutes, or until set and the top is lightly golden.
5. Remove the casserole from the oven and let it cool for 5 minutes.
6. Sprinkle the top with shredded coconut and chopped walnuts or almonds.

Baked Millet Cakes with Pear and Cardamom

 Time:
45 minutes

 Prep Time:
15 minutes

Serving Size:
2 servings

Cook Time:
30 minutes

Each Serving Has:
Calories: 228, Carbohydrates: 39g, Saturated Fat: 0.4g, Protein: 5g, Fat: 7g, Sodium: 62mg, Potassium: 202mg, Fiber: 4g, Sugar: 7g, Vitamin C: 5mg, Calcium: 14mg, Iron: 1mg

Ingredients:
- 1/2 cup [95g] cooked millet, cooled
- 1/2 cup [75g] grated peeled pear
- 1 tbsp ground flaxseed
- 2 tbsp unsweetened oat milk
- 1 tbsp maple syrup
- 1/4 tsp ground cardamom
- 1/4 tsp ground cinnamon
- 1/2 tsp olive oil

Directions:
1. Preheat the oven to 350°F [175°C]. Lightly grease a small baking sheet with olive oil.
2. In a small bowl, whisk together ground flaxseed and oat milk. Let sit for 5 minutes to form a gel-like consistency.
3. In a medium bowl, combine cooked millet, grated pear, maple syrup, ground cardamom, and ground cinnamon.
4. Stir the flaxseed mixture into the millet mixture until fully incorporated and the ingredients are evenly distributed.
5. Divide the mixture into four equal portions and shape into compact patties, about 2½ inches [6.5 cm] in diameter.
6. Place the patties on the prepared baking sheet and bake for 25–30 minutes, flipping them once halfway through, until they are lightly golden and firm.
7. Let cool for 5 minutes before serving warm.

Roasted Carrot and Oat Porridge

🕐	Time: 30 minutes	🍽	Serving Size: 2 bowls
🥗	Prep Time: 10 minutes	👨‍🍳	Cook Time: 20 minutes

Each Serving Has:
Calories: 240, Carbohydrates: 38g, Saturated Fat: 1g, Protein: 6g, Fat: 7g, Sodium: 50mg, Potassium: 400mg, Fiber: 5g, Sugar: 8g, Vitamin C: 6mg, Calcium: 60mg, Iron: 2mg.

Ingredients:
- 1/2 cup [40g] of old-fashioned oats
- 1 cup [240ml] of unsweetened almond milk
- 1/2 cup [120ml] of water
- 1 medium carrot, peeled and grated (about 1/2 cup [50g])
- 1 tbsp of pure maple syrup
- 1/4 tsp of ground cinnamon
- 1/8 tsp of ground nutmeg
- 1 tbsp of unsalted sunflower seeds (for garnish)
- 1/2 tbsp of unsweetened shredded coconut (for garnish)

Directions:
1. Preheat the oven to 375°F. Place the grated carrot on a parchment-lined baking sheet and roast for 10 minutes, stirring halfway through, until lightly caramelized.
2. While the carrot is roasting, combine oats, almond milk, and water in a saucepan. Place over medium heat and stir gently.
3. Add cinnamon and nutmeg to the oat mixture and stir well. Cook for 8-10 minutes, stirring occasionally, until the oats are creamy and the liquid is absorbed.
4. Once the carrots are roasted, stir them into the cooked oats along with the maple syrup. Cook for an additional 2 minutes, allowing the flavors to meld together.
5. Sprinkle each serving with sunflower seeds and shredded coconut.

Quinoa and Poppy Seed Breakfast Bars

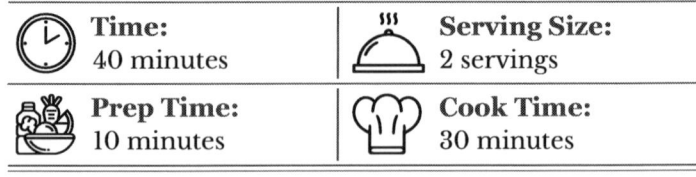

🕐	Time: 40 minutes	🍽	Serving Size: 2 servings
🥗	Prep Time: 10 minutes	👨‍🍳	Cook Time: 30 minutes

Each Serving Has:
Calories: 214, Carbohydrates: 30g, Saturated Fat: 0.6g, Protein: 6g, Fat: 8g, Sodium: 74mg, Potassium: 210mg, Fiber: 4g, Sugar: 7g, Vitamin C: 2mg, Calcium: 54mg, Iron: 2mg

Ingredients:
- 1/2 cup [85g] cooked quinoa, cooled
- 1/4 cup [60ml] unsweetened almond milk
- 1/4 cup [60g] mashed ripe banana
- 2 tbsp grated
- peeled apple
- 1 tbsp maple syrup
- 1 tbsp ground flaxseed
- 1 tbsp poppy seeds
- 1/4 tsp ground cinnamon
- 1/2 tsp olive oil

Directions:
1. Preheat the oven to 350°F [175°C]. Lightly grease a small square baking dish or loaf pan with olive oil.
2. In a large bowl, combine cooked quinoa, mashed banana, grated apple, almond milk, maple syrup, ground flaxseed, poppy seeds, and ground cinnamon. Stir until a uniform batter forms.
3. Pour the mixture into the prepared baking dish and smooth the top evenly with a spatula.
4. Bake for 28–30 minutes, or until the top is firm and lightly golden.
5. Let it cool in the pan for 10 minutes, then slice into two bars. Serve warm.

Spinach and Asparagus Egg Wraps

 Time: 20 minutes

 Serving Size: 2 wraps

 Prep Time: 10 minutes

 Cook Time: 10 minutes

Each Serving Has:

Calories: 190, Carbohydrates: 8g, Saturated Fat: 1g, Protein: 12g, Fat: 12g, Sodium: 140mg, Potassium: 400mg, Fiber: 2g, Sugar: 2g, Vitamin C: 12mg, Calcium: 50mg, Iron: 2mg.

Ingredients:

- 4 large eggs
- 2 tbsp of unsweetened almond milk
- 1/4 tsp of ground turmeric
- 1/4 tsp of dried oregano
- 1/4 tsp of ground black pepper (optional)
- 1 tbsp of olive oil
- 1/2 cup [50g]
- of fresh spinach, chopped
- 1/2 cup [50g] of asparagus spears, trimmed and chopped into 1-inch pieces
- 2 whole-grain tortillas (8 inches)
- 1 tbsp of unsalted sunflower seeds (for garnish)

Directions:

1. In a bowl, whisk together eggs, almond milk, turmeric, oregano, and black pepper (if using). Set aside.
2. Heat 1/2 tbsp olive oil in a non-stick skillet over medium and sauté asparagus for 3–4 minutes until tender.
3. Add spinach to the skillet and cook for 1-2 minutes, stirring frequently, until wilted. Remove the vegetables from the skillet and set aside.
4. Reduce heat to low, add the remaining 1/2 tbsp of olive oil to the skillet. Pour in the egg mixture. Cook for 3-4 minutes, stirring gently until fully cooked but still soft.
5. Warm tortillas in a dry skillet for 30 seconds on each side.
6. Divide the scrambled eggs and vegetables evenly among the tortillas, then roll them tightly into wraps.
7. Sprinkle sunflower seeds over the wraps.

Polenta with Steamed Pears

 Time: 25 minutes

Serving Size: 2 servings

Prep Time: 5 minutes

 Cook Time: 20 minutes

Each Serving Has:

Calories: 210, Carbohydrates: 39g, Saturated Fat: 0.5g, Protein: 4g, Fat: 4g, Sodium: 30mg, Potassium: 250mg, Fiber: 5g, Sugar: 14g, Vitamin C: 8mg, Calcium: 40mg, Iron: 1mg.

Ingredients:

- 1/2 cup [85g] of polenta (coarse cornmeal)
- 2 cups [480ml] of water
- 1 medium pear, peeled, cored, and thinly sliced
- 1/2 tsp of ground cinnamon
- 1/2 tsp of pure vanilla extract
- 1 tbsp of pure maple syrup
- 1/4 tsp of ground nutmeg

Directions:

1. In a saucepan, bring 2 cups of water to a boil. Slowly whisk in polenta, then reduce heat to low. Cook for 15 minutes, stirring frequently, until smooth and thickened.
2. While the polenta is cooking, prepare the pears. Place pear slices in a steamer basket over simmering water. Cover and steam for 5-7 minutes, or until the pears are tender.
3. Once the polenta is cooked, remove from heat and stir in vanilla extract and cinnamon.
4. Arrange the steamed pear slices on top of the polenta.
5. Drizzle each serving with maple syrup and sprinkle with nutmeg.

Pumpkin Spice Oatmeal with Maple Syrup

 **Time:**
15 minutes

 Serving Size:
2 bowls

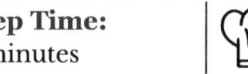 **Prep Time:**
5 minutes

Cook Time:
10 minutes

Each Serving Has:
Calories: 210, Carbohydrates: 38g, Saturated Fat: 0.5g, Protein: 6g, Fat: 4g, Sodium: 40mg, Potassium: 300mg, Fiber: 6g, Sugar: 10g, Vitamin C: 5mg, Calcium: 50mg, Iron: 2mg.

Ingredients:
- 1 cup [80g] of old-fashioned oats
- 1 1/2 cups [360ml] of unsweetened almond milk
- 1/2 cup [120g] of canned pumpkin purée
- 1/2 tsp of ground cinnamon
- 1/4 tsp of ground nutmeg
- 1/8 tsp of ground ginger
- 1 tbsp of pure maple syrup
- 1 tbsp of unsalted pumpkin seeds (for garnish)
- 1/2 tbsp of unsweetened shredded coconut (for garnish)

Directions:
1. In a saucepan, combine oats and almond milk. Place over medium heat and stir gently.
2. Add pumpkin purée, cinnamon, nutmeg, and ginger to the saucepan. Stir well to combine.
3. Cook the mixture for 8-10 minutes, stirring occasionally, until the oats are creamy and the flavors are well combined.
4. Remove the oatmeal from the heat and stir in the maple syrup.
5. Sprinkle each serving with pumpkin seeds and a bit of shredded coconut.

Buckwheat and Banana Muffins

 Time:
30 minutes

 Serving Size:
2 servings

 Prep Time:
10 minutes

 Cook Time:
20 minutes

Each Serving Has:
Calories: 220, Carbohydrates: 36g, Saturated Fat: 0.5g, Protein: 5g, Fat: 6g, Sodium: 50mg, Potassium: 320mg, Fiber: 4g, Sugar: 12g, Vitamin C: 5mg, Calcium: 40mg, Iron: 1.5mg.

Ingredients:
- 1/2 cup [80g] of buckwheat flour
- 1/2 tsp of baking powder
- 1/4 tsp of ground cinnamon
- 1/8 tsp of ground nutmeg
- 1 medium ripe banana, mashed
- 1/4 cup [60ml]
- of unsweetened almond milk
- 1 tbsp of pure maple syrup
- 1 tbsp of unsweetened shredded coconut (for garnish)
- 1 tbsp of unsalted sunflower seeds (for garnish)

Directions:
1. Preheat your oven to 350°F. Line a muffin tin with 4 paper liners or grease lightly with oil.
2. In a bowl, whisk together buckwheat flour, baking powder, cinnamon, and nutmeg until evenly combined.
3. In another bowl, mash banana until smooth, then stir in almond milk and maple syrup until well blended.
4. Gently fold wet ingredients into dry, stirring just until combined. Avoid overmixing for tender muffins.
5. Divide the batter evenly into muffin liners, filling each about two-thirds full.
6. Sprinkle the muffin tops with shredded coconut and sunflower seeds.
7. Bake for 18–20 minutes, or until a toothpick inserted into the center comes out clean.
8. Let the muffins cool for 5 minutes in the tin, then transfer to a wire rack to cool completely.

Rice Flake Cereal with Almond Milk

Time: 10 minutes	**Serving Size:** 2 bowls
Prep Time: 5 minutes	**Cook Time:** 5 minutes

Each Serving Has:
Calories: 190, Carbohydrates: 36g, Saturated Fat: 0.5g, Protein: 4g, Fat: 4g, Sodium: 60mg, Potassium: 120mg, Fiber: 2g, Sugar: 6g, Vitamin C: 2mg, Calcium: 50mg, Iron: 1mg.

Ingredients:
- 1 cup [50g] of rice flakes
- 1 cup [240ml] of unsweetened almond milk
- 1/4 tsp of ground cinnamon
- 1 tsp of pure maple syrup
- 1/2 medium banana, thinly sliced
- 1 tbsp of unsweetened shredded coconut (for garnish)
- 1 tbsp of unsalted pumpkin seeds (for garnish)

Directions:
1. In a saucepan, warm almond milk over medium heat. Add cinnamon and maple syrup, stirring until well combined. Heat for 2-3 minutes, but do not boil.
2. Place the rice flakes in a mixing bowl. Pour the warmed almond milk mixture over the rice flakes and stir gently to combine. Let the mixture sit for 1-2 minutes to soften the flakes.
3. Slice the banana thinly and layer the slices evenly over the prepared rice flake cereal.
4. Sprinkle with unsweetened shredded coconut and unsalted pumpkin seeds.

Soft Oatmeal Pancakes with Blueberries

Time: 20 minutes	**Serving Size:** 2 pancakes
Prep Time: 10 minutes	**Cook Time:** 10 minutes

Each Serving Has:
Calories: 250, Carbohydrates: 38g, Saturated Fat: 0.5g, Protein: 6g, Fat: 6g, Sodium: 190mg, Potassium: 200mg, Fiber: 5g, Sugar: 8g, Vitamin C: 5mg, Calcium: 60mg, Iron: 1.5mg

Ingredients:
- 1/2 cup [40g] old-fashioned oats
- 1/2 cup [75g] whole wheat flour
- 1 tsp baking powder
- 1/4 tsp baking soda
- 1/4 tsp ground cinnamon
- 1 large egg
- 1/2 cup [120ml]
- unsweetened almond milk
- 1 tbsp pure maple syrup
- 1/2 tsp vanilla extract
- 1/2 cup [75g] fresh blueberries (divided)
- 1 tbsp avocado oil or canola oil

Directions:
1. Blend oats into a flour-like consistency, then transfer to a bowl. Add whole wheat flour, baking powder, baking soda, and cinnamon. Whisk to combine.
2. In another bowl, whisk the egg until frothy. Stir in almond milk, maple syrup, and vanilla extract until combined.
3. Gradually mix wet and dry ingredients until smooth, avoiding overmixing. Fold in half of the blueberries.
4. Heat a non-stick skillet over medium heat and greas it with avocado oil. Pour 1/4 cup of batter per pancake onto the hot skillet.
5. Cook for 2–3 minutes, until bubbles form and the edges are set. Flip and cook for more 2 minutes, until golden brown and cooked through.
6. Transfer pancakes to a plate and repeat with the remaining batter.
7. Top with the remaining blueberries and serve.

Banana and Oat Breakfast Cookies

Time: 25 minutes	Serving Size: 2 servings
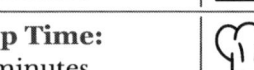 Prep Time: 10 minutes	Cook Time: 15 minutes

Each Serving Has:
Calories: 180, Carbohydrates: 30g, Saturated Fat: 0.5g, Protein: 4g, Fat: 5g, Sodium: 30mg, Potassium: 200mg, Fiber: 4g, Sugar: 10g, Vitamin C: 2mg, Calcium: 20mg, Iron: 1mg.

Ingredients:
- 1 medium ripe banana, mashed
- 1/2 cup [40g] of old-fashioned oats
- 1 tbsp of ground flaxseed
- 1 tbsp of pure maple syrup
- 1/4 tsp of ground cinnamon
- 1/4 tsp of ground nutmeg
- 1 tbsp of unsweetened shredded coconut (for garnish)

Directions:
1. Preheat your oven to 350°F. Line a baking sheet with parchment paper.
2. In a mixing bowl, mash banana until smooth. Add oats, flaxseed, maple syrup, cinnamon, and nutmeg. Stir until well combined.
3. Scoop 1–2 tablespoons of the mixture, roll into a ball, and place on the baking sheet. Flatten gently with a spoon to form cookies. Repeat with the remaining mixture to make 6 cookies.
4. Sprinkle the cookies with shredded coconut.
5. Bake in the preheated oven for 12-15 minutes, or until the cookies are firm and lightly golden.
6. Allow the cookies to cool on the baking sheet for 5 minutes before transferring them to a wire rack to cool completely.

Buckwheat and Coconut Milk Porridge with Pears

Time: 20 minutes	Serving Size: 2 bowls
Prep Time: 5 minutes	Cook Time: 15 minutes

Each Serving Has:
Calories: 290, Carbohydrates: 48g, Saturated Fat: 3g, Protein: 6g, Fat: 7g, Sodium: 40mg, Potassium: 340mg, Fiber: 6g, Sugar: 12g, Vitamin C: 6mg, Calcium: 40mg, Iron: 1.7mg

Ingredients:
- 1/2 cup [85g] raw buckwheat groats
- 1 cup [240ml] unsweetened coconut milk
- 1/2 cup [120ml] water
- 1 tbsp pure maple syrup
- 1/4 tsp ground cinnamon
- 1 medium ripe pear, diced
- 1 tbsp unsweetened shredded coconut, toasted
- 1 tbsp chopped unsalted almonds or walnuts (for garnish)

Directions:
1. Rinse buckwheat groats under cold running water in a fine-mesh strainer to remove any residue.
2. In a saucepan, combine the rinsed buckwheat groats, coconut milk, and water. Bring to a gentle boil over medium heat.
3. Reduce heat to low, add cinnamon, and cover. Simmer for 10-12 minutes, stirring occasionally, until tender and mostly absorbed.
4. Dice the pear and set aside. For extra flavor, toast shredded coconut in a dry skillet over medium heat for 2–3 minutes, stirring until golden.
5. Once the buckwheat porridge is ready, remove it from the heat and stir in maple syrup.
6. Top with pear, shredded coconut, and a sprinkle of almonds or walnuts, if desired.

Soft Polenta with Pumpkin Puree

Time: 20 minutes	Serving Size: 2 servings
Prep Time: 5 minutes	Cook Time: 15 minutes

Each Serving Has:

Calories: 190, Carbohydrates: 32g, Saturated Fat: 1g, Protein: 4g, Fat: 4g, Sodium: 40mg, Potassium: 350mg, Fiber: 5g, Sugar: 8g, Vitamin C: 6mg, Calcium: 30mg, Iron: 1mg.

Ingredients:
- 1/2 cup [85g] of polenta (coarse cornmeal)
- 2 cups [480ml] of unsweetened almond milk
- 1/2 cup [120g] of canned pumpkin puree
- 1/4 tsp of ground cinnamon
- 1/4 tsp of ground nutmeg
- 1 tbsp of pure maple syrup
- 1 tbsp of unsweetened shredded coconut (for garnish)
- 1/2 tbsp of unsalted pumpkin seeds (for garnish)

Directions:
1. In a saucepan, bring almond milk to a gentle boil over medium heat. Gradually whisk in the polenta to prevent lumps from forming.
2. Reduce the heat to low and continue to cook the polenta, stirring frequently, for 10-12 minutes, or until it reaches a creamy consistency.
3. Once the polenta is cooked, stir in pumpkin puree, cinnamon, nutmeg, and maple syrup. Mix until all the ingredients are well incorporated and heated through.
4. Remove from heat. Garnish with a sprinkle of shredded coconut and pumpkin seeds.

Zucchini and Sweet Potato Breakfast Hash

Time: 25 minutes	Serving Size: 2 plates
Prep Time: 10 minutes	Cook Time: 15 minutes

Each Serving Has:

Calories: 210, Carbohydrates: 36g, Saturated Fat: 0.5g, Protein: 4g, Fat: 5g, Sodium: 40mg, Potassium: 450mg, Fiber: 6g, Sugar: 8g, Vitamin C: 10mg, Calcium: 40mg, Iron: 1mg.

Ingredients:
- 1 medium sweet potato, peeled and diced (about 1 cup [150g])
- 1 medium zucchini, diced (about 1 cup [150g])
- 1 tbsp of olive oil
- 1/2 tsp of ground turmeric
- 1/4 tsp of ground cinnamon
- 1/4 tsp of dried thyme
- 1 tbsp of pure maple syrup
- 1 tbsp of unsalted sunflower seeds (for garnish)

Directions:
1. Heat the olive oil in a large, non-stick skillet over medium heat.
2. Add sweet potato to the skillet and sauté for 8–10 minutes, stirring occasionally, until softened and golden.
3. Add zucchini to the skillet, stir to combine, and cook for 5 more minutes, stirring occasionally, until tender.
4. Sprinkle turmeric, cinnamon, and thyme over the vegetables. Stir to evenly coat the sweet potato and zucchini with the spices.
5. Drizzle maple syrup over the hash, toss gently, and cook for 1-2 more minutes to meld the flavors.
6. Remove the skillet from heat and garnish with sunflower seeds.

Applesauce Pancakes with Chia Seeds

 Time:
20 minutes

 Serving Size:
2 servings

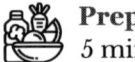 **Prep Time:**
5 minutes

 Cook Time:
15 minutes

Each Serving Has:
Calories: 200, Carbohydrates: 35g, Saturated Fat: 0.5g, Protein: 5g, Fat: 4g, Sodium: 100mg, Potassium: 150mg, Fiber: 6g, Sugar: 8g, Vitamin C: 3mg, Calcium: 50mg, Iron: 1.5mg.

Ingredients:
- 1/2 cup [60g] of whole wheat flour
- 1/4 cup [30g] of rolled oats
- 1/2 tsp of baking powder
- 1/4 tsp of ground cinnamon
- 1 tbsp of chia seeds
- 1/2 cup [120ml] of unsweetened applesauce
- 1/4 cup [60ml] of unsweetened almond milk
- 1/2 tsp of pure vanilla extract
- 1 tbsp of pure maple syrup (optional)
- 1/2 tbsp of olive oil for cooking

Directions:
1. In a bowl, combine whole wheat flour, oats, baking powder, cinnamon, and chia seeds. Stir to evenly distribute the dry ingredients.
2. In a separate bowl, whisk together applesauce, almond milk, vanilla extract, and maple syrup (if using).
3. Gradually add the wet ingredients to the dry ingredients, stirring gently until just combined. Avoid over mixing to ensure fluffy pancakes.
4. Heat a non-stick skillet over medium heat and lightly coat with olive oil.
5. Pour 1/4 cup of batter onto the skillet for each pancake. Cook for 2-3 minutes, until bubbles form and edges set. Flip carefully and cook for another 2 minutes, until golden brown.
6. Repeat with the remaining batter, adding more oil to the skillet as needed.
7. Top with a drizzle of pure maple syrup or a sprinkle of extra chia seeds, if desired.

Roasted Beet and Oatmeal Bowl

 Time:
30 minutes

 Serving Size:
2 bowls

 Prep Time:
10 minutes

 Cook Time:
20 minutes

Each Serving Has:
Calories: 220, Carbohydrates: 38g, Saturated Fat: 0.5g, Protein: 6g, Fat: 5g, Sodium: 40mg, Potassium: 300mg, Fiber: 7g, Sugar: 8g, Vitamin C: 8mg, Calcium: 50mg, Iron: 2mg.

Ingredients:
- 1 small beet, peeled and diced (about 1/2 cup [75g])
- 1/2 cup [40g] of old-fashioned oats
- 1 cup [240ml] of unsweetened almond milk
- 1/4 tsp of ground cinnamon
- 1/4 tsp of ground
- nutmeg
- 1 tbsp of pure maple syrup
- 1 tbsp of unsalted sunflower seeds (for garnish)
- 1 tbsp of unsweetened shredded coconut (for garnish)

Directions:
1. Preheat the oven to 375°F. Spread beets on a parchment-lined baking sheet and roast for 15 minutes, stirring halfway through, until tender and lightly caramelized.
2. While the beet is roasting, combine oats and almond milk in a saucepan. Place over medium heat and stir gently.
3. Add cinnamon and nutmeg to the saucepan, stirring to combine. Cook for 8-10 minutes, stirring occasionally, until the oats are creamy and cooked through.
4. Once the beets are roasted, fold them into the oatmeal with maple syrup. Cook for 1-2 more minutes to combine the flavors.
5. For added texture and nutrition, sprinkle each bowl with sunflower seeds and shredded coconut.

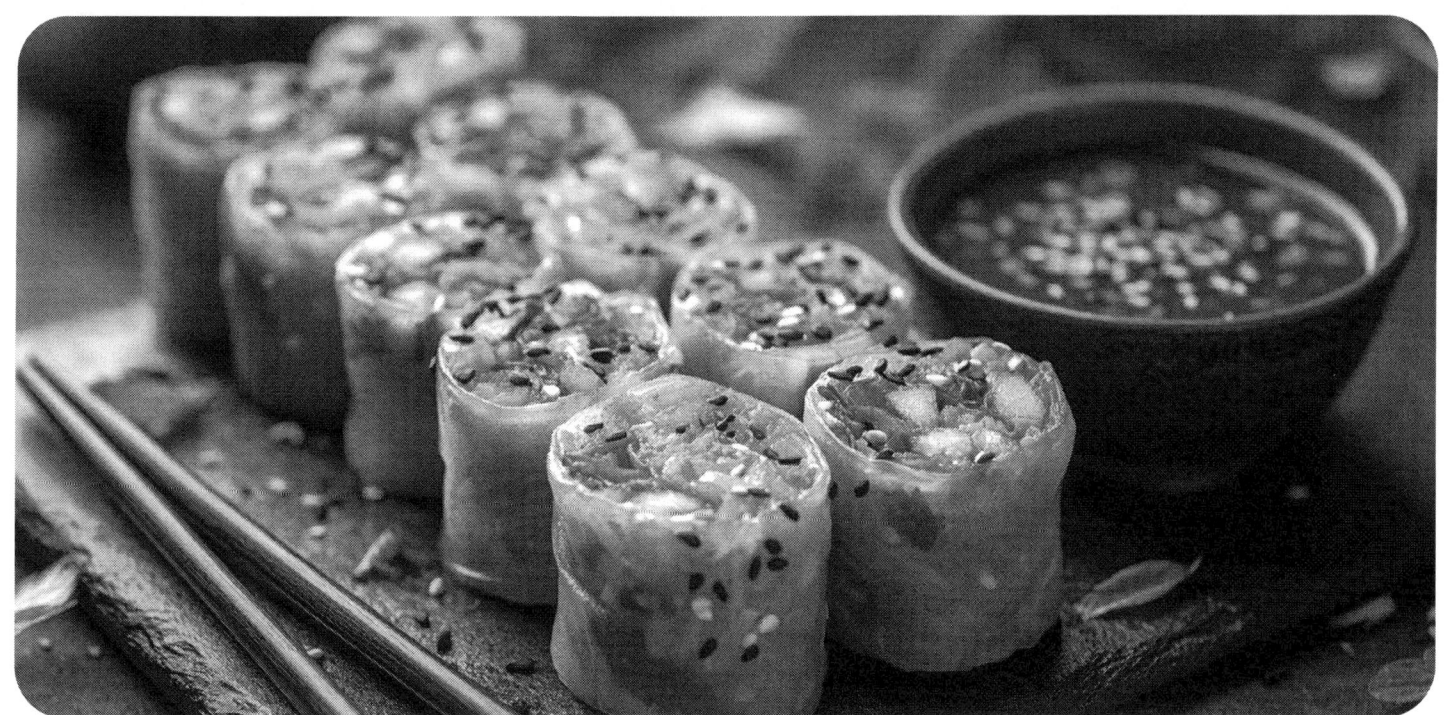

Chapter 3: Snacks and Appetizers

Baked Zucchini Sticks with Basil Yogurt Dip

 Time: 30 minutes

 Serving Size: 2 plates

 Prep Time: 10 minutes

Cook Time: 20 minutes

Each Serving Has:
Calories: 160, Carbohydrates: 12g, Saturated Fat: 1g, Protein: 6g, Fat: 8g, Sodium: 120mg, Potassium: 400mg, Fiber: 3g, Sugar: 4g, Vitamin C: 10mg, Calcium: 60mg, Iron: 1mg.

Ingredients:
For the Zucchini Sticks:
- 1 medium zucchini, cut into sticks (about 3 inches long)
- 1/4 cup [30g] of whole wheat breadcrumbs
- 1/4 tsp of ground turmeric
- 1/4 tsp of dried oregano
- 1 tbsp of olive oil

For the Basil Yogurt Dip:
- 1/2 cup [120g] of low-fat, lactose-free yogurt
- 1 tbsp of fresh basil, finely chopped
- 1/4 tsp of garlic powder
- 1/4 tsp of pure maple syrup (optional)

Directions:
1. Preheat your oven to 400°F. Line a baking sheet with parchment paper.
2. In a bowl, mix breadcrumbs, turmeric, and oregano.
3. Coat the zucchini sticks with olive oil, then roll in the breadcrumb mixture until evenly coated. Arrange them in a single layer on the prepared baking sheet.
4. Bake the zucchini sticks for 18-20 minutes, flipping them halfway through, until golden brown and crispy.
5. While the zucchini bakes, prepare the basil yogurt dip. In a bowl, combine yogurt, basil, garlic powder, and maple syrup (if desired). Mix well and set aside.
6. Remove the zucchini sticks from the oven and let them cool for 2-3 minutes.
7. Serve the baked zucchini sticks warm with the basil yogurt dip on the side.

Roasted Chickpeas with Dill and Olive Oil

 Time:
35 minutes

 Serving Size:
2 bowls

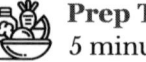 **Prep Time:**
5 minutes

Cook Time:
30 minutes

Each Serving Has:
Calories: 180, Carbohydrates: 25g, Saturated Fat: 1g, Protein: 7g, Fat: 6g, Sodium: 80mg, Potassium: 210mg, Fiber: 6g, Sugar: 2g, Vitamin C: 3mg, Calcium: 40mg, Iron: 1.5mg.

Ingredients:
• 1 cup [150g] of cooked chickpeas, rinsed and patted dry
• 1 tbsp of olive oil
• 1/2 tsp of dried dill
• 1/4 tsp of garlic powder
• 1/4 tsp of ground turmeric
• 1/8 tsp of ground cumin
• 1/8 tsp of sea salt (optional)

Directions:
1. Preheat your oven to 375°F. Line a baking sheet with parchment paper.
2. Place the rinsed and patted-dry chickpeas in a medium bowl. Drizzle with olive oil and toss to coat evenly.
3. In a bowl, mix dill, garlic powder, turmeric, cumin, and sea salt (if using). Sprinkle the spice mixture over the chickpeas and toss until the chickpeas are fully coated.
4. Spread the seasoned chickpeas in a single layer on the prepared baking sheet.
5. Roast in the oven for 25-30 minutes, stirring halfway through, until the chickpeas are golden brown and crispy.
6. Remove the chickpeas from the oven and let them cool for 5 minutes.

Steamed Edamame with Parsley

 Time:
15 minutes

 Serving Size:
2 small bowls

 Prep Time:
5 minutes

 Cook Time:
10 minutes

Each Serving Has:
Calories: 120, Carbohydrates: 10g, Saturated Fat: 0.5g, Protein: 10g, Fat: 4g, Sodium: 25mg, Potassium: 300mg, Fiber: 5g, Sugar: 1g, Vitamin C: 10mg, Calcium: 40mg, Iron: 1.8mg.

Ingredients:
• 1 cup [150g] of frozen edamame in pods
• 1 tbsp of olive oil
• 1 tbsp of fresh parsley, finely chopped
• 1/4 tsp of garlic powder
• 1/4 tsp of ground turmeric
• 1/8 tsp of sea salt (optional)

Directions:
1. Bring a medium pot of water to a boil. Add the frozen edamame and cook for 5 minutes, or until the pods are tender but still firm. Drain and set aside.
2. While the edamame is steaming, prepare the seasoning. In a bowl, combine olive oil, chopped parsley, garlic powder, and turmeric. Mix well to form a fragrant dressing.
3. Place the cooked edamame in a mixing bowl. Pour the parsley and olive oil mixture over the edamame, tossing to ensure the pods are evenly coated.
4. Sprinkle a pinch of sea salt over the edamame, if desired, and toss again.

Sweet Potato Wedges with Oregano

 Time:
30 minutes

 Prep Time:
10 minutes

Serving Size:
2 plates

Cook Time:
20 minutes

Each Serving Has:
Calories: 190, Carbohydrates: 34g, Saturated Fat: 0.5g, Protein: 3g, Fat: 5g, Sodium: 40mg, Potassium: 450mg, Fiber: 5g, Sugar: 8g, Vitamin C: 10mg, Calcium: 40mg, Iron: 1mg.

Ingredients:
- 1 medium sweet potato, scrubbed and cut into wedges (about 1 cup [150g])
- 1 tbsp of olive oil
- 1/2 tsp of dried oregano
- 1/4 tsp of garlic powder
- 1/4 tsp of ground paprika
- 1/8 tsp of sea salt (optional)

Directions:
1. Preheat your oven to 400°F. Line a baking sheet with parchment paper.
2. In a bowl, combine the sweet potato with olive oil. Toss to coat evenly.
3. Sprinkle oregano, garlic powder, paprika, and sea salt (if using) over the sweet potato wedges. Toss again to ensure the wedges are well coated with the seasoning.
4. Arrange the sweet potato wedges in a single layer on the prepared baking sheet, ensuring they do not overlap for even cooking.
5. Bake in the preheated oven for 18-20 minutes, flipping the wedges halfway through, until they are golden brown and crispy on the edges.
6. Remove the wedges from the oven and let them cool for 2-3 minutes.

White Bean and Basil Dip with Rice Crackers

 Time:
10 minutes

 Prep Time:
10 minutes

Serving Size:
2 servings

Cook Time:
0 minutes

Each Serving Has:
Calories: 194, Carbohydrates: 28g, Saturated Fat: 0.7g, Protein: 7g, Fat: 6g, Sodium: 160mg, Potassium: 320mg, Fiber: 5g, Sugar: 1g, Vitamin C: 3mg, Calcium: 52mg, Iron: 2mg

Ingredients:
- 3/4 cup [130g] rinsed and drained canned white beans
- 1 tbsp chopped fresh basil
- 1 tbsp unsweetened oat
- milk
- 1 tbsp olive oil
- 1/8 tsp ground turmeric
- 12 pieces [30g] plain unsalted rice crackers

Directions:
1. In a medium bowl, mash drained white beans with a fork until mostly smooth, leaving some small chunks for texture.
2. Stir in chopped basil, oat milk, olive oil, and ground turmeric, mixing until well combined and creamy.
3. Serve the dip evenly divided between two plates, accompanied by plain unsalted rice crackers.
4. Enjoy immediately, or refrigerate the dip in an airtight container for up to 24 hours and serve chilled.

Pumpkin Seed and Flax Energy Bars

 Time:
20 minutes

 Serving Size:
2 bars

 Prep Time:
10 minutes

 Cook Time:
10 minutes

Each Serving Has:
Calories: 210, Carbohydrates: 22g, Saturated Fat: 0.5g, Protein: 6g, Fat: 9g, Sodium: 20mg, Potassium: 120mg, Fiber: 6g, Sugar: 10g, Vitamin C: 1mg, Calcium: 40mg, Iron: 1.8mg.

Ingredients:
- 1/4 cup [30g] of unsalted pumpkin seeds
- 1/4 cup [30g] of rolled oats
- 1 tbsp of ground flaxseed
- 1/4 cup [60g] of unsweetened applesauce
- 1 tbsp of pure maple syrup
- 1/4 tsp of ground cinnamon
- 1/4 tsp of ground nutmeg

Directions:
1. Preheat your oven to 325°F. Line a small baking dish (approximately 6x6 inches) with parchment paper.
2. In a mixing bowl, combine pumpkin seeds, oats, flaxseed, cinnamon, and nutmeg. Stir to evenly distribute the dry ingredients.
3. Add applesauce and maple syrup to the dry mixture. Stir until all ingredients are well combined and the mixture becomes sticky.
4. Transfer the mixture to the prepared baking dish. Using the back of a spoon, press it down evenly to form a compact layer.
5. Bake in the preheated oven for 8-10 minutes, or until the edges are lightly golden. Remove from the oven and let it cool for 10 minutes in the dish.
6. Once cooled, lift the parchment paper to remove the bar layer from the dish. Cut into 4 equal-sized bars.

Carrot and Zucchini Muffins

 Time:
35 minutes

Serving Size:
2 muffins

 Prep Time:
10 minutes

Cook Time:
25 minutes

Each Serving Has:
Calories: 160, Carbohydrates: 22g, Saturated Fat: 0.5g, Protein: 4g, Fat: 6g, Sodium: 70mg, Potassium: 250mg, Fiber: 4g, Sugar: 6g, Vitamin C: 6mg, Calcium: 50mg, Iron: 1.2mg.

Ingredients:
- 1/2 cup [60g] of whole wheat flour
- 1/4 tsp of baking soda
- 1/4 tsp of baking powder
- 1/4 tsp of ground cinnamon
- 1/4 tsp of ground nutmeg
- 1/4 cup [30g] of grated carrot
- 1/4 cup [30g] of grated zucchini
- 1 tbsp of ground flaxseed
- 1 tbsp of pure maple syrup
- 1/4 cup [60ml] of unsweetened almond milk
- 1 tbsp of olive oil
- 1/4 tsp of pure vanilla extract

Directions:
1. Preheat your oven to 350°F. Line a muffin tin with 4 paper liners or lightly grease the cups with oil.
2. In a mixing bowl, whisk together the whole wheat flour, baking soda, baking powder, cinnamon, and nutmeg.
3. In another bowl, combine carrot, zucchini, flaxseed, maple syrup, almond milk, olive oil, and vanilla extract. Stir well.
4. Gradually fold the wet ingredients into the dry, stirring gently until just combined. Avoid overmixing.
5. Evenly fill muffin cups two-thirds full with batter.
6. Bake for 20-25 minutes, or until a toothpick inserted into the center comes out clean.
7. Cool the muffins in the tin for 5 minutes, then transfer to a wire rack to cool completely.

Roasted Beet Chips with Olive Oil

Time: 30 minutes	Serving Size: 2 servings
Prep Time: 10 minutes	Cook Time: 20 minutes

Each Serving Has:
Calories: 100, Carbohydrates: 14g, Saturated Fat: 0.5g, Protein: 2g, Fat: 3g, Sodium: 60mg, Potassium: 300mg, Fiber: 3g, Sugar: 8g, Vitamin C: 5mg, Calcium: 15mg, Iron: 0.8mg.

Ingredients:
• 1 medium beet, peeled and thinly sliced (about 1 cup [150g])
• 1 tbsp of olive oil
• 1/4 tsp of dried oregano
• 1/4 tsp of garlic powder
• 1/8 tsp of sea salt (optional)

Directions:
1. Preheat your oven to 375°F. Line a baking sheet with parchment paper.
2. Using a sharp knife or mandoline, slice the beet as thinly as possible for even cooking.
3. In a bowl, toss the beet slices with olive oil until evenly coated.
4. Sprinkle oregano, garlic powder, and sea salt (if using) over the beet slices. Toss again to evenly distribute the seasoning.
5. Arrange the beet slices in a single layer on the prepared baking sheet, ensuring they do not overlap.
6. Bake in the preheated oven for 18-20 minutes, flipping the slices halfway through, until they are crisp and slightly golden. Keep a close eye to prevent burning, as thin slices can cook quickly.
7. Remove the beet chips from the oven and let them cool for 5 minutes on the baking sheet.

Roasted Fennel Slices

Time: 40 minutes	Serving Size: 2 servings
Prep Time: 10 minutes	Cook Time: 30 minutes

Each Serving Has:
Calories: 132, Carbohydrates: 11g, Saturated Fat: 1g, Protein: 2g, Fat: 10g, Sodium: 42mg, Potassium: 457mg, Fiber: 4g, Sugar: 5g, Vitamin C: 13mg, Calcium: 66mg, Iron: 1mg

Ingredients:
• 1 1/2 cups [180g] thinly sliced fresh fennel bulb
• 1 tbsp chopped fresh thyme
• 1 tbsp olive oil
• 1/4 tsp sea salt (optional)

Directions:
1. Preheat the oven to 375°F [190°C]. Line a small baking sheet with parchment paper.
2. In a large bowl, toss thinly sliced fennel bulb with olive oil, chopped thyme, and sea salt (if using), ensuring the fennel is evenly coated.
3. Spread the fennel slices in a single layer on the prepared baking sheet.
4. Roast for 30 minutes, turning the slices halfway through, until the fennel is tender and the edges are lightly golden.
5. Let cool slightly before serving warm.

Wild Rice and Cucumber Salad Cups

 Time:
25 minutes

 Serving Size:
2 cups

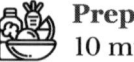 **Prep Time:**
10 minutes

 Cook Time:
15 minutes

Each Serving Has:

Calories: 160, Carbohydrates: 28g, Saturated Fat: 0.5g, Protein: 4g, Fat: 4g, Sodium: 20mg, Potassium: 200mg, Fiber: 3g, Sugar: 2g, Vitamin C: 5mg, Calcium: 20mg, Iron: 1.2mg.

Ingredients:

- 1/4 cup [50g] of uncooked wild rice
- 1 medium cucumber, sliced into thick rounds (about 12 slices)
- 1 tbsp of olive oil
- 1 tsp of rice vinegar
- 1/2 tsp of pure maple syrup
- 2 tbsp of fresh parsley, finely chopped
- 1/4 tsp of ground ginger

Directions:

1. Cook rice according to the package instructions, using about 3/4 cup [180ml] of water. Once cooked, drain any excess water and let the rice cool slightly.
2. While the rice cooks, slice the cucumber into thick rounds and use a small spoon to scoop out the centers, creating cups without scooping through the bottom.
3. In a bowl, whisk together olive oil, rice vinegar, maple syrup, ginger, and half of the parsley to create a light dressing.
4. Once rice has cooled, combine it with the dressing, stirring to coat the grains evenly.
5. Spoon the dressed rice mixture into the cucumber cups, packing it lightly to fill each one.
6. Garnish each cucumber cup with the remaining parsley.

Baked Carrot and Quinoa Balls

 Time:
40 minutes

 Serving Size:
2 servings

 Prep Time:
15 minutes

 Cook Time:
25 minutes

Each Serving Has:

Calories: 198, Carbohydrates: 26g, Saturated Fat: 0.5g, Protein: 6g, Fat: 8g, Sodium: 88mg, Potassium: 340mg, Fiber: 4g, Sugar: 4g, Vitamin C: 5mg, Calcium: 42mg, Iron: 2mg

Ingredients:

- 1/2 cup [85g] cooked quinoa, cooled
- 1/2 cup [60g] grated peeled carrot
- 1 tbsp chopped fresh parsley
- 1 tbsp ground flaxseed
- 2 tbsp unsweetened almond milk
- 1 tbsp olive oil
- 1 tbsp grated zucchini
- 1/4 tsp dried thyme
- 1/2 tsp olive oil

Directions:

1. Preheat the oven to 375°F [190°C]. Lightly grease a baking sheet with olive oil.
2. In a small bowl, whisk together ground flaxseed and almond milk. Let sit for 5 minutes to thicken into a flax "egg."
3. In a large bowl, combine cooked quinoa, grated carrot, chopped parsley, grated zucchini, and dried thyme.
4. Stir in the flax mixture and olive oil, mixing until all ingredients are well combined and the mixture holds together.
5. Using your hands, form the mixture into 8 small, equal-sized balls and place them evenly spaced on the prepared baking sheet.
6. Bake for 25 minutes, turning the balls halfway through, until they are lightly golden and firm to the touch.
7. Let cool for 5 minutes before serving warm.

Apple and Cinnamon Snack Bites

 Time:
15 minutes

 Serving Size:
2 servings

 Prep Time:
10 minutes

 Cook Time:
5 minutes

Each Serving Has:

Calories: 120, Carbohydrates: 20g, Saturated Fat: 0.5g, Protein: 2g, Fat: 4g, Sodium: 15mg, Potassium: 150mg, Fiber: 3g, Sugar: 12g, Vitamin C: 4mg, Calcium: 20mg, Iron: 0.6mg.

Ingredients:

- 1 medium apple, peeled, cored, and grated (about 1/2 cup [75g])
- 1/4 cup [20g] of rolled oats
- 1 tbsp of ground flaxseed
- 1 tbsp of
- unsweetened applesauce
- 1/4 tsp of ground cinnamon
- 1/4 tsp of ground nutmeg
- 1 tsp of pure maple syrup (optional)

Directions:

1. In a bowl, combine apple, oats, flaxseed, applesauce, cinnamon, and nutmeg. Mix thoroughly to form a sticky mixture.
2. If you prefer a sweeter snack, add maple syrup and mix well to evenly distribute.
3. Using your hands, form the mixture into small, bite-sized balls (about 1 inch in diameter). You should get about 6-8 bites.
4. Heat a non-stick skillet over low heat and lightly toast the snack bites for 1-2 minutes on each side to bring out the flavors and firm them slightly. Alternatively, you can enjoy them raw without toasting.
5. Allow the bites to cool slightly before serving.

Millet and Zucchini Fritters

 Time:
40 minutes

Serving Size:
2 servings

 Prep Time:
15 minutes

Cook Time:
25 minutes

Each Serving Has:

Calories: 212, Carbohydrates: 28g, Saturated Fat: 0.7g, Protein: 5g, Fat: 9g, Sodium: 98mg, Potassium: 326mg, Fiber: 4g, Sugar: 3g, Vitamin C: 11mg, Calcium: 34mg, Iron: 1mg

Ingredients:

- 1/2 cup [95g] cooked millet, cooled
- 1/2 cup [60g] grated zucchini, squeezed dry
- 1/4 cup [30g] grated peeled carrot
- 1 tbsp chopped
- fresh parsley
- 1 tbsp ground flaxseed
- 2 tbsp unsweetened oat milk
- 1/4 tsp dried thyme
- 1 tbsp olive oil

Directions:

1. Preheat the oven to 375°F [190°C]. Line a baking sheet with parchment paper and set aside.
2. In a small bowl, whisk together ground flaxseed and oat milk. Let sit for 5 minutes to form a thick flax mixture.
3. In a medium bowl, combine the cooked millet, grated zucchini, carrots, chopped parsley, and dried thyme. Stir until the vegetables are evenly distributed.
4. Add the flax mixture to the bowl and mix thoroughly until a soft, moldable dough forms.
5. Shape the mixture into 6 small patties and place them evenly spaced on the prepared baking sheet.
6. Lightly brush the tops of the fritters with half of the olive oil. Bake for 15 minutes.
7. Remove the tray from the oven, carefully flip the fritters, and brush the other sides with the remaining olive oil. Return the dish to the oven and bake for an additional 10 minutes, until golden and firm.
8. Let cool for 5 minutes before serving warm.

Roasted Parsnip Sticks with Thyme

⏱ **Time:** 30 minutes	🍽 **Serving Size:** 2 plates
🥗 **Prep Time:** 10 minutes	👨‍🍳 **Cook Time:** 20 minutes

Each Serving Has:
Calories: 110, Carbohydrates: 18g, Saturated Fat: 0.5g, Protein: 2g, Fat: 4g, Sodium: 40mg, Potassium: 300mg, Fiber: 5g, Sugar: 5g, Vitamin C: 10mg, Calcium: 30mg, Iron: 0.7mg.

Ingredients:
- 2 medium parsnips, peeled and cut into sticks (about 1 cup [150g])
- 1 tbsp of olive oil
- 1/2 tsp of dried thyme
- 1/4 tsp of garlic powder
- 1/8 tsp of sea salt (optional)

Directions:
1. Preheat your oven to 400°F. Line a baking sheet with parchment paper.
2. Place the parsnip sticks in a bowl. Drizzle with olive oil and toss to coat evenly.
3. Sprinkle thyme, garlic powder, and sea salt (if using) over the parsnip sticks. Toss again to ensure the sticks are well coated with the seasoning.
4. Arrange the seasoned parsnip sticks in a single layer on the prepared baking sheet, ensuring they do not overlap for even cooking.
5. Roast in the preheated oven for 18-20 minutes, flipping halfway through, until the parsnip sticks are golden brown and tender.
6. Remove the roasted parsnip sticks from the oven and let them cool for 2-3 minutes before serving.

Soft Baked Pear and Oat Bars

⏱ **Time:** 35 minutes	🍽 **Serving Size:** 2 servings
🥗 **Prep Time:** 10 minutes	👨‍🍳 **Cook Time:** 25 minutes

Each Serving Has:
Calories: 214, Carbohydrates: 33g, Saturated Fat: 0.5g, Protein: 5g, Fat: 7g, Sodium: 58mg, Potassium: 245mg, Fiber: 4g, Sugar: 10g, Vitamin C: 4mg, Calcium: 40mg, Iron: 1mg

Ingredients:
- 1/2 cup [50g] rolled oats
- 1/2 cup [75g] grated peeled pear
- 2 tbsp mashed ripe banana
- 1 tbsp maple syrup
- 1 tbsp unsweetened almond milk
- 1 tbsp ground flaxseed
- 1/2 tsp ground cinnamon
- 1/2 tsp olive oil

Directions:
1. Preheat the oven to 350°F [175°C]. Lightly grease a small baking dish with olive oil.
2. In a medium bowl, combine rolled oats, grated pear, mashed banana, maple syrup, almond milk, ground flaxseed, and ground cinnamon. Mix until all ingredients are thoroughly incorporated.
3. Transfer the mixture into the prepared baking dish and press it down evenly with a spatula to form a compact layer.
4. Bake for 25 minutes, or until the top is lightly golden and the center is set.
5. Allow the bars to cool in the dish for 10 minutes before slicing into two bars.
6. Serve warm.

Cucumber and Spinach Pinwheels

	Time: 15 minutes		Serving Size: 2 servings
	Prep Time: 15 minutes		Cook Time: 0 minutes

Each Serving Has:

Calories: 130, Carbohydrates: 15g, Saturated Fat: 1g, Protein: 4g, Fat: 6g, Sodium: 80mg, Potassium: 250mg, Fiber: 3g, Sugar: 2g, Vitamin C: 5mg, Calcium: 40mg, Iron: 0.8mg.

Ingredients:

- 2 small whole wheat tortillas
- 1/4 cup [60g] of low-fat cream cheese
- 1/2 cup [15g] of fresh spinach, finely chopped
- 1/4 cup [30g] of grated cucumber (excess water squeezed out)
- 1/4 tsp of garlic powder
- 1/4 tsp of dried dill
- 1/8 tsp of sea salt (optional)

Directions:

1. Lay tortillas flat on a clean surface. Spread an equal amount of cream cheese evenly across each tortilla.
2. In a bowl, mix spinach, cucumber, garlic powder, dill, and sea salt (if using). Stir until well combined.
3. Spread the spinach and cucumber mixture evenly over the cream cheese layer on each tortilla.
4. Roll the tortillas tightly into logs. Use a sharp knife to slice each log into 1-inch pinwheels.

Steamed Green Beans with Herb Dressing

	Time: 15 minutes		Serving Size: 2 plates
	Prep Time: 5 minutes		Cook Time: 10 minutes

Each Serving Has:

Calories: 90, Carbohydrates: 10g, Saturated Fat: 0.5g, Protein: 2g, Fat: 6g, Sodium: 15mg, Potassium: 200mg, Fiber: 4g, Sugar: 3g, Vitamin C: 10mg, Calcium: 40mg, Iron: 1mg.

Ingredients:

- 2 cups [150g] of fresh green beans, trimmed
- 1 tbsp of olive oil
- 1/4 tsp of garlic powder
- 1 tsp of fresh
- parsley, finely chopped
- 1/2 tsp of dried thyme
- 1/8 tsp of sea salt (optional)

Directions:

1. Fill a medium saucepan with 1 inch of water and bring it to a boil. Place a steamer basket over the saucepan, and add the trimmed green beans. Cover and steam for 7-10 minutes, or until the beans are tender but still crisp.
2. While the beans steam, prepare the herb dressing. In a bowl, whisk together olive oil, garlic powder, parsley, thyme, and sea salt (if using).
3. Once the green beans are cooked, transfer them to a serving dish. Drizzle the herb dressing evenly over the beans and toss gently to coat.

Rice Cakes with Pumpkin Spread

⏱ **Time:** 10 minutes	🍽 **Serving Size:** 2 rice cakes
🥗 **Prep Time:** 10 minutes	👨‍🍳 **Cook Time:** 0 minutes

Each Serving Has:

Calories: 140, Carbohydrates: 24g, Saturated Fat: 0.5g, Protein: 2g, Fat: 4g, Sodium: 10mg, Potassium: 200mg, Fiber: 3g, Sugar: 3g, Vitamin C: 4mg, Calcium: 20mg, Iron: 0.8mg.

Ingredients:

- 4 plain rice cakes
- 1/2 cup [120g] of canned pumpkin puree (unsweetened)
- 1/2 tsp of ground cinnamon
- 1/4 tsp of ground nutmeg
- 1 tsp of pure maple syrup
- 1/4 tsp of vanilla extract
- 1 tbsp of unsalted pumpkin seeds (for garnish)

Directions:

1. In a mixing bowl, combine pumpkin puree, cinnamon, nutmeg, maple syrup, and vanilla extract. Stir until the mixture is smooth and well blended.
2. Spread an equal amount of the pumpkin mixture onto each rice cake, covering the surface evenly.
3. Sprinkle pumpkin seeds over the pumpkin spread for added texture and nutrition.

Chia Coconut Cups with Poached Apple

⏱ **Time:** 20 minutes	🍽 **Serving Size:** 2 servings
🥗 **Prep Time:** 10 minutes	👨‍🍳 **Cook Time:** 10 minutes

Each Serving Has:

Calories: 198, Carbohydrates: 28g, Saturated Fat: 3g, Protein: 4g, Fat: 9g, Sodium: 42mg, Potassium: 310mg, Fiber: 7g, Sugar: 13g, Vitamin C: 5mg, Calcium: 128mg, Iron: 2mg

Ingredients:

- 1/4 cup [60ml] unsweetened coconut milk beverage
- 3/4 cup [180ml] unsweetened almond milk
- 3 tbsp chia seeds
- 1 tbsp maple syrup
- 1/2 tsp vanilla extract
- 1 large apple, peeled, cored, and diced
- 1/4 cup [60ml] water
- 1/4 tsp ground cinnamon

Directions:

1. In a small bowl, whisk together coconut milk beverage, almond milk, chia seeds, maple syrup, and vanilla extract until well combined.
2. Let the mixture sit at room temperature for 10 minutes, then stir again to prevent clumping. Cover and refrigerate for at least 2 hours, or until the mixture has thickened to a pudding consistency.
3. While the pudding chills, combine diced apple, water, and ground cinnamon in a small saucepan.
4. Bring to a gentle simmer over low heat and cook for 10 minutes, stirring occasionally, until the apple is soft and the liquid is mostly absorbed.
5. Allow the poached apple to cool to room temperature, then divide evenly between two serving cups.
6. Spoon the chilled chia pudding over the apples and serve immediately.

Carrot and Celery Sticks with Yogurt Dill Dip

Time: 10 minutes	**Serving Size:** 2 small plates
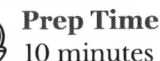 **Prep Time:** 10 minutes	**Cook Time:** 0 minutes

Each Serving Has:

Calories: 90, Carbohydrates: 10g, Saturated Fat: 0.5g, Protein: 4g, Fat: 3g, Sodium: 50mg, Potassium: 300mg, Fiber: 3g, Sugar: 4g, Vitamin C: 8mg, Calcium: 80mg, Iron: 0.5mg.

Ingredients:

- 2 medium carrots, peeled and cut into sticks (about 1 cup [120g])
- 2 celery stalks, cut into sticks (about 1 cup [100g])
- 1/4 cup [60g] of plain low-fat yogurt
- 1/2 tsp of dried dill
- 1/4 tsp of garlic powder
- 1 tsp of lemon juice (optional)
- 1/8 tsp of sea salt (optional)

Directions:

1. Prepare the carrot and celery sticks by washing, peeling (carrots only), and cutting them into evenly sized sticks for easy dipping. Arrange them on a serving plate.
2. In a bowl, combine yogurt, dill, garlic powder, lemon juice (if using), and sea salt (if desired). Stir well until the mixture is smooth and the seasonings are evenly distributed.
3. Transfer the yogurt dill dip to a small serving bowl. Place it on the plate alongside the carrot and celery sticks.

Roasted Cauliflower Bites with Garlic-Free Sauce

Time: 30 minutes	**Serving Size:** 2 plates
Prep Time: 10 minutes	**Cook Time:** 20 minutes

Each Serving Has:

Calories: 110, Carbohydrates: 12g, Saturated Fat: 0.5g, Protein: 3g, Fat: 6g, Sodium: 40mg, Potassium: 200mg, Fiber: 4g, Sugar: 2g, Vitamin C: 30mg, Calcium: 20mg, Iron: 0.7mg.

Ingredients:

- 2 cups [200g] of cauliflower florets
- 1 tbsp of olive oil
- 1/2 tsp of smoked paprika
- 1/4 tsp of ground cumin
- 1/8 tsp of sea salt (optional)
- For the Sauce:
- 1/4 cup [60g] of plain low-fat yogurt
- 1 tsp of fresh lemon juice (optional)
- 1/2 tsp of dried parsley
- 1/4 tsp of ground turmeric

Directions:

1. Preheat your oven to 400°F. Line a baking sheet with parchment paper.
2. In a bowl, toss cauliflower with olive oil, smoked paprika, cumin, and sea salt (if using). Mix until the cauliflower is evenly coated.
3. Spread the seasoned cauliflower in a single layer on the prepared baking sheet. Roast in the preheated oven for 18-20 minutes, flipping halfway through, until the cauliflower is tender and slightly caramelized.
4. While the cauliflower roasts, prepare the garlic-free sauce. In a bowl, whisk together yogurt, lemon juice (if using), parsley, and turmeric until smooth and well combined.
5. Transfer the roasted cauliflower bites to a serving plate and serve warm with the garlic-free yogurt sauce on the side for dipping.

Baked Plantain Chips with Sea Salt

Time: 25 minutes	Serving Size: 2 servings
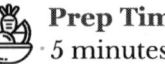 Prep Time: 5 minutes	Cook Time: 20 minutes

Each Serving Has:
Calories: 150, Carbohydrates: 32g, Saturated Fat: 1g, Protein: 1g, Fat: 2g, Sodium: 50mg, Potassium: 450mg, Fiber: 2g, Sugar: 10g, Vitamin C: 10mg, Calcium: 10mg, Iron: 0.3mg.

Ingredients:
- 1 medium plantain, peeled and thinly sliced
- 1 tbsp of olive oil
- 1/4 tsp of sea salt
- 1/4 tsp of smoked paprika (optional)

Directions:
1. Preheat your oven to 375°F. Line a baking sheet with parchment paper.
2. Slice plantain into thin, even rounds using a sharp knife or mandoline slicer.
3. In a mixing bowl, toss the plantain slices with olive oil, ensuring each slice is lightly coated. Sprinkle it with sea salt and smoked paprika (if using) for added flavor.
4. Arrange the plantain slices in a single layer on the prepared baking sheet, ensuring they do not overlap.
5. Bake in the preheated oven for 18-20 minutes, flipping the slices halfway through, until they are golden brown and crisp.
6. Remove the chips from the oven and let them cool for 5 minutes before serving.

Kohlrabi Sticks with Yogurt Dip

Time: 20 minutes	Serving Size: 2 servings
Prep Time: 10 minutes	Cook Time: 10 minutes

Each Serving Has:
Calories: 112, Carbohydrates: 14g, Saturated Fat: 1g, Protein: 5g, Fat: 5g, Sodium: 88mg, Potassium: 514mg, Fiber: 5g, Sugar: 6g, Vitamin C: 49mg, Calcium: 120mg, Iron: 1mg

Ingredients:
- 2 cups [240g] peeled and sliced into sticks kohlrabi
- 1/2 cup [120g] unsweetened low-fat plain yogurt
- 1 tbsp chopped
- fresh dill
- 1 tbsp unsweetened almond milk
- 1/2 tsp olive oil
- 1/4 tsp ground cumin

Directions:
1. Fill a saucepan with 1 inch [2.5 cm] of water and bring to a gentle boil. Place the kohlrabi sticks in a steamer basket over the boiling water.
2. Cover and steam the kohlrabi for 8–10 minutes, or until just tender when pierced with a fork. Remove from heat and let cool slightly.
3. In a small bowl, combine plain yogurt, chopped dill, almond milk, olive oil, and ground cumin. Stir until smooth and creamy.
4. Divide the steamed kohlrabi sticks evenly between two plates and serve with the dill yogurt dip on the side. Serve warm.

Rice Paper Rolls

Time: 35 minutes	Serving Size: 2 servings
Prep Time: 20 minutes	Cook Time: 15 minutes

Each Serving Has:

Calories: 202, Carbohydrates: 34g, Saturated Fat: 0.5g, Protein: 5g, Fat: 5g, Sodium: 48mg, Potassium: 372mg, Fiber: 3g, Sugar: 2g, Vitamin C: 11mg, Calcium: 49mg, Iron: 2mg

Ingredients:

- 1/2 cup [95g] rinsed millet
- 1 1/4 cups [300ml] water
- 1/2 cup [10g] chopped fresh spinach
- 1/2 cup [50g]
- julienned peeled cucumber
- 1 tbsp chopped fresh basil
- 1 tsp olive oil
- 6 round rice paper sheets [about 22cm diameter each]

Directions:

1. In a small saucepan, combine rinsed millet and water. Bring to a boil over medium heat.
2. Reduce the heat to low, cover, and simmer for 12–15 minutes, or until the millet is soft and most of the liquid has been absorbed. Remove from heat and let it sit, covered, for 5 minutes.
3. Gently fluff the millet with a fork, then stir in the chopped spinach, basil, and olive oil. Let the mixture cool slightly to room temperature.
4. Fill a wide, shallow dish with warm water. Dip one rice paper sheet into the water for 5–10 seconds, until it becomes pliable but not overly soft.
5. Lay the softened sheet flat on a clean surface. Place a spoonful of the millet mixture in the center, then top with julienned cucumber.
6. Fold the sides of the rice paper over the filling, then roll tightly from the bottom to form a neat roll.
7. Repeat this process with the remaining rice paper sheets and filling to make a total of six rolls.
8. Serve immediately.

Polenta Squares with Roasted Sunchokes and Parsnips

Time: 50 minutes	Serving Size: 2 servings
Prep Time: 15 minutes	Cook Time: 35 minutes

Each Serving Has:

Calories: 310, Carbohydrates: 42g, Saturated Fat: 2g, Protein: 6g, Fat: 13g, Sodium: 180mg, Potassium: 650mg, Fiber: 5g, Sugar: 4g, Vitamin C: 12mg, Calcium: 45mg, Iron: 1.5mg

Ingredients:

- 1/2 cup [80g] ground yellow cornmeal (polenta)
- 2 cups [480ml] water
- 2/3 cup [85g] sunchokes (Jerusalem artichokes), peeled and cubed
- 3/4 cup [85g]
- parsnips, peeled and cut into matchsticks
- 1 tbsp olive oil (+ 1/2 tsp extra for greasing)
- 1/2 tsp fresh thyme, finely chopped
- 1/4 tsp sea salt

Directions:

1. Preheat the oven to 400°F [200°C]. Line a baking sheet with parchment paper and grease a loaf pan with olive oil.
2. Toss sunchokes and parsnips with olive oil on a baking sheet.
3. Roast the vegetables for 20 minutes, flipping halfway, until tender and golden.
4. Boil the water in a saucepan and slowly whisk in cornmeal, stirring to prevent lumps.
5. Simmer on low for 8-10 minutes, or until the polenta is thick. Remove from heat, stir in chopped thyme and pour it into the loaf pan.
6. Let the polenta cool at room temperature for 10 minutes, then refrigerate it for at least 15 minutes, or until it is firm
7. Once set, cut the polenta into squares, then sear them in a nonstick skillet over medium heat for 3 minutes per side, or until golden.
8. Divide the polenta and roasted vegetables between two plates. Serve warm.

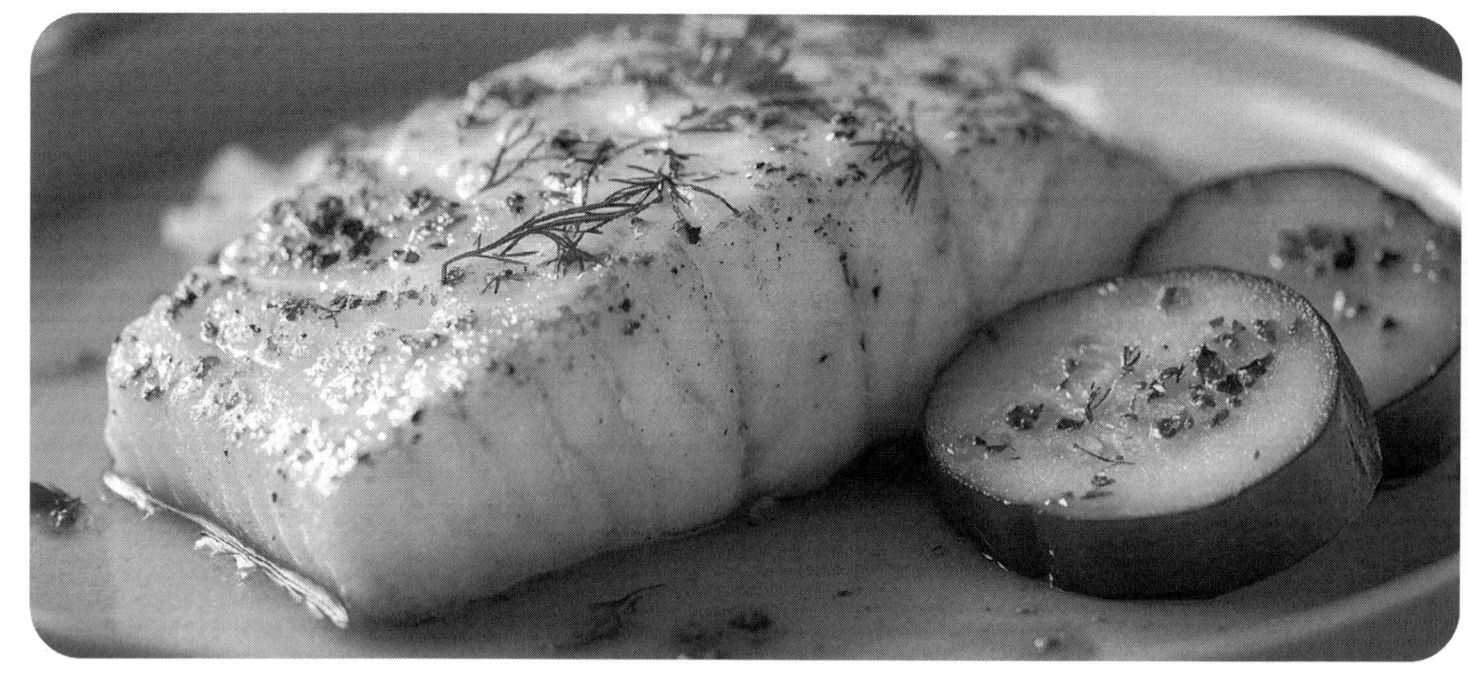

Chapter 4: Lunch

Chicken Millet Patties with Dill Yogurt

Time: 45 minutes	Serving Size: 2 servings
Prep Time: 20 minutes	Cook Time: 25 minutes

Each Serving Has:
Calories: 284, Carbohydrates: 19g, Saturated Fat: 1g, Protein: 22g, Fat: 14g, Sodium: 132mg, Potassium: 410mg, Fiber: 2g, Sugar: 2g, Vitamin C: 3mg, Calcium: 68mg, Iron: 2mg

Ingredients:
- 1/2 cup [95g] cooked and cooled millet
- 1/2 cup [100g] chopped cooked skinless chicken breast
- 1/4 cup [30g] grated zucchini, squeezed dry
- 1 tbsp chopped fresh parsley
- 1 tbsp ground flaxseed
- 2 tbsp unsweetened almond milk
- 1/4 tsp dried thyme
- 1/2 tsp olive oil
- 1/2 cup [120g] unsweetened low-fat plain yogurt
- 1 tbsp chopped fresh dill
- 1 tbsp unsweetened almond milk

Directions:
1. Preheat the oven to 375°F [190°C]. Lightly grease a baking sheet with olive oil.
2. In a small bowl, whisk together ground flaxseed and almond milk. Let sit for 5 minutes to thicken.
3. In a large bowl, combine cooked millet, chopped cooked chicken breast, grated zucchini, chopped parsley, and dried thyme. Mix well to incorporate.
4. Add the flax mixture to the bowl and stir until the ingredients bind together.
5. Form the mixture into 6 small patties and place them evenly spaced on the prepared baking sheet.
6. Bake for 25 minutes, flipping the patties halfway through, until they are firm and lightly golden.
7. While the patties bake, prepare the sauce by whisking together plain yogurt, chopped dill, and almond milk in a small bowl until smooth.
8. Divide the patties between two plates and serve with the dill yogurt sauce on the side.

Quinoa and Broccoli Bowl with Olive Oil

 Time:
25 minutes

 Serving Size:
2 bowls

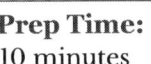 **Prep Time:**
10 minutes

 Cook Time:
15 minutes

Each Serving Has:
Calories: 230, Carbohydrates: 35g, Saturated Fat: 1g, Protein: 8g, Fat: 7g, Sodium: 50mg, Potassium: 400mg, Fiber: 5g, Sugar: 3g, Vitamin C: 70mg, Calcium: 50mg, Iron: 2mg.

Ingredients:
- 1/2 cup [90g] of quinoa, rinsed
- 1 cup [240ml] of water
- 1 cup [150g] of broccoli florets, steamed
- 1/4 cup [60g] of grated zucchini
- 2 tbsp of extra virgin olive oil
- 1 tsp of fresh parsley, chopped (for garnish)
- 1/8 tsp of sea salt (optional)

Directions:
1. Rinse the quinoa under cold running water to remove bitterness. In a saucepan, combine the quinoa and water. Bring to a boil, then reduce the heat to low, cover, and simmer for 12-15 minutes, until the quinoa is tender and the water is absorbed.
2. While the quinoa cooks, steam broccoli for about 5 minutes, or until tender but still vibrant green.
3. In a mixing bowl, combine quinoa, broccoli, and zucchini.
4. Drizzle the olive oil over the quinoa mixture, and sprinkle with sea salt (if using). Toss gently to combine and evenly coat the ingredients.
5. Garnish with fresh parsley.

Lentil and Sweet Potato Salad with Parsley

 Time:
35 minutes

 Serving Size:
2 bowls

 Prep Time:
10 minutes

Cook Time:
25 minutes

Each Serving Has:
Calories: 310, Carbohydrates: 50g, Saturated Fat: 1g, Protein: 12g, Fat: 8g, Sodium: 55mg, Potassium: 670mg, Fiber: 12g, Sugar: 6g, Vitamin C: 25mg, Calcium: 60mg, Iron: 4mg.

Ingredients:
- 1/2 cup [100g] of dry green lentils
- 1 medium sweet potato, peeled and diced (about 8 oz [227g])
- 1 tbsp of extra virgin olive oil
- 1/2 tsp of ground cumin
- 1/8 tsp of ground black pepper (optional)
- 1/8 tsp of sea salt
- 1/4 cup [15g] of fresh parsley, chopped
- 1/4 cup [60ml] of plain unsweetened yogurt (optional)

Directions:
1. Rinse the lentils under cold water and place them in a medium saucepan. Cover with water, bring to a boil, then reduce to a simmer and cook for 20-25 minutes, until tender but not mushy. Drain and set aside.
2. While the lentils cook, preheat the oven to 375°F. Spread the sweet potato on a baking sheet. Drizzle with 1/2 tbsp of olive oil and sprinkle with cumin and black pepper (if using). Toss to coat, then roast for 20-25 minutes, flipping halfway through, until tender and lightly browned.
3. In a mixing bowl, combine the cooked lentils, roasted sweet potato, and chopped parsley. Drizzle with the remaining olive oil and gently toss to combine. Add sea salt.
4. If using yogurt, add a dollop on top of each serving for a creamy finish.

Zucchini Noodles with Basil Pesto

 Time:
20 minutes

 **Serving Size:**
2 bowls

 Prep Time:
10 minutes

 Cook Time:
10 minutes

Each Serving Has:
Calories: 210, Carbohydrates: 12g, Saturated Fat: 2g, Protein: 6g, Fat: 16g, Sodium: 90mg, Potassium: 500mg, Fiber: 4g, Sugar: 6g, Vitamin C: 20mg, Calcium: 40mg, Iron: 2mg.

Ingredients:
- 2 medium zucchini (about 10 oz [283g])
- 1/4 cup [60ml] of extra virgin olive oil
- 1/4 cup [15g] of fresh basil leaves
- 1 tbsp of raw sunflower seeds
- 1 tbsp of unsweetened plain yogurt
- 1/8 tsp of sea salt
- 2 tbsp of grated reduced-fat Parmesan cheese

Directions:
1. Use a spiralizer or julienne peeler to create zucchini noodles. Set the noodles on a paper towel to remove excess moisture.
2. In a blender or food processor, combine basil leaves, sunflower seeds, olive oil, and yogurt. Blend until smooth, pausing to scrape down the sides as needed. Add Parmesan and sea salt, then pulse until well combined.
3. Heat a non-stick skillet over medium heat. Add the zucchini noodles and sauté for 2-3 minutes until just tender but still slightly firm.
4. Remove the skillet from heat and toss the noodles with the prepared basil pesto until evenly coated.
5. Garnish with a sprinkle of grated Parmesan.

Steamed Cod with Carrot Puree and Quinoa

 Time:
45 minutes

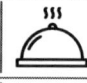 **Serving Size:**
2 servings

 Prep Time:
15 minutes

 Cook Time:
30 minutes

Each Serving Has:
Calories: 310, Carbohydrates: 28g, Saturated Fat: 1g, Protein: 28g, Fat: 10g, Sodium: 78mg, Potassium: 708mg, Fiber: 4g, Sugar: 6g, Vitamin C: 10mg, Calcium: 41mg, Iron: 2mg

Ingredients:
- 2 fillets [200g] fresh cod, skinless and boneless
- 1/2 cup [85g] rinsed quinoa
- 1 cup [240ml] water
- 1 1/2 cups [210g] peeled and chopped carrots
- 1/2 cup [120ml] unsweetened almond milk
- 1 tsp chopped fresh parsley
- 1 tbsp olive oil
- 1/8 tsp ground turmeric
- 1/8 tsp ground coriander
- 1/8 tsp dried oregano

Directions:
1. Preheat the oven to 400°F [200°C]. Line a baking sheet with parchment paper and grease a loaf pan with olive oil.
2. Toss sunchokes and parsnips with olive oil on a baking sheet.
3. Roast the vegetables for 20 minutes, flipping halfway, until tender and golden.
4. Boil the water in a saucepan and slowly whisk in cornmeal, stirring to prevent lumps.
5. Simmer on low for 8-10 minutes, or until the polenta is thick. Remove from heat, stir in chopped thyme and pour it into the loaf pan.
6. Let the polenta cool at room temperature for 10 minutes, then refrigerate it for at least 15 minutes, or until it is firm
7. Once set, cut the polenta into squares, then sear them in a nonstick skillet over medium heat for 3 minutes per side, or until golden.
8. Divide the polenta and roasted vegetables between two plates. Serve warm.

Roasted Beetroot and Cauliflower Bowl

Time: 35 minutes	Serving Size: 2 bowls
Prep Time: 10 minutes	Cook Time: 25 minutes

Each Serving Has:

Calories: 240, Carbohydrates: 28g, Saturated Fat: 1g, Protein: 6g, Fat: 10g, Sodium: 140mg, Potassium: 710mg, Fiber: 7g, Sugar: 10g, Vitamin C: 55mg, Calcium: 45mg, Iron: 2.5mg.

Ingredients:

- 1 medium beetroot, peeled and diced (approx. 6 oz [170g])
- 1 small cauliflower, cut into florets (approx. 8 oz [227g])
- 2 tbsp of olive oil
- 1/4 tsp of ground cumin
- 1/4 tsp of ground coriander
- 1/8 tsp of sea salt
(optional)
- 1/4 cup [60ml] of plain unsweetened yogurt
- 1 tbsp of tahini
- 1 tbsp of fresh parsley, chopped (for garnish)
- 1/4 cup [30g] of cooked quinoa
- 1 tbsp of toasted sunflower seeds (for garnish)

Directions:

1. Preheat the oven to 400°F. Line a baking sheet with parchment paper.
2. In a mixing bowl, toss beetroot and cauliflower with olive oil, cumin, coriander, and sea salt (if using) until evenly coated.
3. Spread the vegetables on the prepared baking sheet in a single layer. Roast in the oven for 20–25 minutes, turning halfway through, until tender and slightly caramelized.
4. While the vegetables roast, whisk yogurt and tahini until smooth.
5. Serve quinoa topped with beetroot and cauliflower, then drizzle with dressing.
6. Garnish with parsley and sunflower seeds.

Turkey and Millet Stuffed Cabbage Rolls

Time: 1 hour	Serving Size: 2 servings
Prep Time: 25 minutes	Cook Time: 35 minutes

Each Serving Has:

Calories: 312, Carbohydrates: 26g, Saturated Fat: 1g, Protein: 26g, Fat: 10g, Sodium: 72mg, Potassium: 628mg, Fiber: 5g, Sugar: 4g, Vitamin C: 36mg, Calcium: 68mg, Iron: 3mg

Ingredients:

- 4 large outer leaves [200g] green cabbage
- 1/2 cup [85g] rinsed millet
- 1 cup [240ml] water
- 1/2 cup [75g] grated zucchini
- 1/2 cup [60g]
chopped cooked carrots
- 6 oz [170g] ground lean turkey
- 1 tbsp chopped fresh parsley
- 1/2 tsp dried thyme
- 1 tbsp olive oil

Directions:

1. Bring water to a gentle boil. Blanch the cabbage leaves for 3 minutes until pliable. Drain and let them cool.
2. Combine millet and water in a saucepan. Bring to a boil, reduce heat to low, cover, and simmer 15 minutes until tender and water is absorbed. Remove from heat and let stand, covered.
3. Heat olive oil in a nonstick skillet over medium-low heat. Sauté grated zucchini and chopped carrots for 5 minutes until softened. Transfer to a bowl.
4. Add cooked millet, ground turkey, chopped parsley, and dried thyme to the vegetable mixture. Stir to combine.
5. Lay each cabbage leaf flat and place half the turkey mixture in the center. Fold in sides and roll tightly to seal.
6. Place rolls seam-side down in a steamer basket. Steam over simmering water for 15–18 minutes, until turkey is cooked and rolls are tender.
7. Transfer to plates and serve.

Lentil and Roasted Fennel Casserole

| 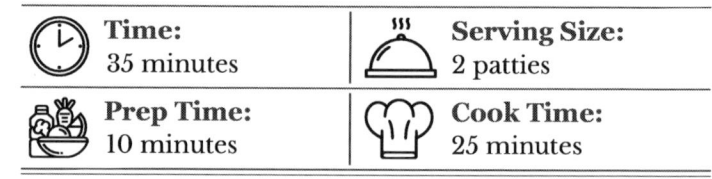 **Time:** 1 hour | **Serving Size:** 2 servings |
| **Prep Time:** 20 minutes | **Cook Time:** 40 minutes |

Each Serving Has:

Calories: 318, Carbohydrates: 42g, Saturated Fat: 1g, Protein: 16g, Fat: 10g, Sodium: 90mg, Potassium: 780mg, Fiber: 15g, Sugar: 6g, Vitamin C: 23mg, Calcium: 85mg, Iron: 5mg

Ingredients:
- 1/2 cup [100g] rinsed green lentils
- 1 1/2 cups [360ml] water
- 1 cup [120g] thinly sliced fennel bulb
- 1/2 cup [60g] chopped zucchini
- 1/2 cup [60g] chopped peeled carrot
- 1/4 cup [40g] chopped cooked sweet potato
- 1 tbsp chopped fresh parsley
- 1/2 tsp dried thyme
- 1 tbsp olive oil

Directions:
1. Preheat the oven to 375°F [190°C]. Line a baking sheet with parchment paper.
2. Spread thinly sliced fennel bulb evenly on the prepared baking sheet. Drizzle with 1/2 tablespoon of olive oil and roast for 20 minutes until lightly browned and tender. Set aside.
3. In a small saucepan, combine green lentils and water. Bring to a boil, then reduce the heat to low, cover, and simmer for 25 minutes, or until tender. Drain any excess liquid and set aside.
4. In a medium skillet, heat the remaining 1/2 tablespoon of olive oil over medium heat. Sauté chopped zucchini and carrot for 5 minutes until softened.
5. In a large bowl, combine cooked lentils, roasted fennel, sautéed zucchini and carrot, mashed sweet potato, chopped parsley, and dried thyme. Stir until thoroughly mixed.
6. Transfer the lentil mixture to a small casserole dish and spread evenly.
7. Bake for 15 minutes until the top is lightly golden and the casserole is heated through.
8. Let rest for 5 minutes before serving.

Baked Turkey Patties with Sweet Potato Mash

| **Time:** 35 minutes | **Serving Size:** 2 patties |
| **Prep Time:** 10 minutes | **Cook Time:** 25 minutes |

Each Serving Has:

Calories: 340, Carbohydrates: 40g, Saturated Fat: 1g, Protein: 25g, Fat: 8g, Sodium: 85mg, Potassium: 750mg, Fiber: 6g, Sugar: 7g, Vitamin C: 20mg, Calcium: 50mg, Iron: 2mg.

Ingredients:
- 6 oz [170g] of ground turkey
- 1/4 cup [40g] of finely chopped zucchini
- 1 tbsp of fresh parsley, finely chopped
- 1/2 tsp of ground coriander
- 1/8 tsp of sea salt (optional)
- 1 tbsp of olive oil
- 1 medium sweet potato (about 10 oz [280g]), peeled and cubed
- 1/4 cup [60ml] of unsweetened almond milk
- 1/2 tsp of ground cinnamon

Directions:
1. Preheat the oven to 375°F.
2. In a mixing bowl, combine the ground turkey, zucchini, parsley, coriander, and sea salt (if using). Mix thoroughly.
3. Shape the mixture into four equal patties and place them on a parchment-lined baking sheet.
4. Lightly brush the patties with olive oil and bake for 20–25 minutes, flipping halfway, until golden and cooked through
5. While the patties bake, boil the sweet potato over medium heat for 12–15 minutes until tender.
6. Drain the sweet potato, transfer to a bowl, add almond milk and cinnamon, then mash until smooth and creamy.
7. Serve the baked turkey patties with sweet potato mash.

Lentil and Spinach Casserole

 Time:
40 minutes

 Serving Size:
2 bowls

 Prep Time:
10 minutes

 Cook Time:
30 minutes

Each Serving Has:

Calories: 320, Carbohydrates: 45g, Saturated Fat: 1g, Protein: 18g, Fat: 6g, Sodium: 140mg, Potassium: 750mg, Fiber: 12g, Sugar: 5g, Vitamin C: 20mg, Calcium: 90mg, Iron: 6mg.

Ingredients:

- 1/2 cup [100g] of dried green lentils
- 1 1/4 cups [300ml] of low-sodium vegetable broth
- 1 medium carrot, finely diced
- 1 celery stalk, finely diced
- 1/2 cup [80g] of finely chopped zucchini
- 1/4 cup [40g] of finely diced onion (optional, depending on sensitivity)
- 1 cup [30g] of fresh spinach, chopped
- 1/4 tsp of ground cumin
- 1/4 tsp of ground coriander
- 1 tbsp of olive oil
- 2 tbsp of unsweetened almond milk
- 1 tbsp of fresh parsley, finely chopped (for garnish)

Directions:

1. Preheat the oven to 375°F.
2. Rinse and drain the lentils. Combine with vegetable broth in a saucepan, bring to a boil, then simmer for 15–20 minutes until tender but not mushy.
3. Heat olive oil in a skillet over medium heat. Sauté carrot, celery, zucchini, and onion (if using) for 5–7 minutes until softened.
4. Combine cooked lentils with sautéed vegetables, then add spinach, cumin, coriander, and almond milk. Mix well.
5. Spread mixture in a baking dish and bake for 10–15 minutes until heated through and golden on top.
6. Cool the casserole for 5 minutes, then garnish with chopped parsley before serving.

Poached White Fish with Steamed Vegetables

 Time:
30 minutes

Serving Size:
2 plates

 Prep Time:
10 minutes

Cook Time:
20 minutes

Each Serving Has:

Calories: 250, Carbohydrates: 18g, Saturated Fat: 1g, Protein: 28g, Fat: 6g, Sodium: 140mg, Potassium: 850mg, Fiber: 5g, Sugar: 6g, Vitamin C: 30mg, Calcium: 60mg, Iron: 2mg.

Ingredients:

- 2 fillets of white fish (e.g., cod, haddock) (8 oz [227g] each)
- 1 1/2 cups [350ml] of low-sodium vegetable broth
- 1 bay leaf
- 1 small zucchini, sliced into rounds
- 1 cup [150g] of broccoli florets
- 1 medium carrot, cut into thin strips
- 1 tbsp of olive oil
- 1 tsp of fresh dill, chopped (for garnish)
- 1/2 tsp of ground coriander
- 1/4 tsp of ground turmeric
- 1/8 tsp of salt (optional)

Directions:

1. In a skillet, pour the vegetable broth and add the bay leaf. Bring the broth to a gentle simmer over medium heat.
2. Place the fish fillets into the simmering broth. Cover and poach for 10–12 minutes, or until the fish flakes easily with a fork. Remove the fish and set aside.
3. While the fish is poaching, prepare the vegetables. In a steamer or a large saucepan fitted with a steaming basket, arrange the zucchini, broccoli, and carrot. Steam for 8–10 minutes until tender but still slightly crisp.
4. Drizzle the steamed vegetables with olive oil, and season with coriander and turmeric. Toss gently to coat evenly.
5. Plate the poached fish alongside the steamed vegetables. Garnish with fresh dill.

Wild Rice and Mushroom Bowl with Parsley

 Time:
35 minutes

 Serving Size:
2 bowls

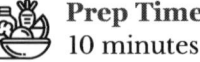 **Prep Time:**
10 minutes

 Cook Time:
25 minutes

Each Serving Has:
Calories: 280, Carbohydrates: 42g, Saturated Fat: 1g, Protein: 8g, Fat: 6g, Sodium: 120mg, Potassium: 510mg, Fiber: 5g, Sugar: 3g, Vitamin C: 12mg, Calcium: 35mg, Iron: 2mg.

Ingredients:
- 1/2 cup [100g] of wild rice
- 1 1/4 cups [300ml] of low-sodium vegetable broth
- 1 tsp of olive oil
- 1/2 cup [50g] of sliced cremini mushrooms
- 1/2 cup [50g] of diced zucchini
- 1/4 cup [30g] of diced yellow bell pepper
- 1 tsp of fresh parsley, chopped
- 1/4 tsp of ground turmeric
- 1/4 tsp of ground coriander
- 1/4 of tsp salt (optional)
- 1 tbsp of unsweetened almond milk (optional)

Directions:
1. Rinse the rice under cold water and drain. In a saucepan, bring the vegetable broth to a boil. Add the rice, reduce the heat to low, cover, and simmer for 20–25 minutes until the rice is tender and the broth is absorbed.
2. In a skillet, heat the olive oil over medium heat. Add the mushrooms and sauté for 3 minutes until slightly softened.
3. Add the zucchini and bell pepper to the skillet. Sprinkle it with turmeric and coriander. Sauté for another 5–7 minutes until the vegetables are tender.
4. Remove the skillet from the heat and stir in parsley.
5. Divide the cooked wild rice between two bowls. Top each bowl with the sautéed vegetables and garnish with a drizzle of almond milk, if desired.

Roasted Carrot and Barley Salad

 Time:
40 minutes

 Serving Size:
2 bowls

 Prep Time:
10 minutes

 Cook Time:
30 minutes

Each Serving Has:
Calories: 250, Carbohydrates: 42g, Saturated Fat: 1g, Protein: 7g, Fat: 5g, Sodium: 120mg, Potassium: 490mg, Fiber: 6g, Sugar: 5g, Vitamin C: 15mg, Calcium: 40mg, Iron: 2mg.

Ingredients:
- 1/2 cup [100g] of pearl barley
- 1 1/4 cups [300ml] of low-sodium vegetable broth
- 2 medium carrots, sliced lengthwise
- 1 tsp of olive oil
- 1/4 tsp of ground coriander
- 1/4 tsp of ground turmeric
- 1/8 tsp of salt
- (optional)
- 1/2 cup [50g] of baby spinach leaves
- 1/4 cup [20g] of fresh parsley, chopped
- 1 tbsp of pumpkin seeds (for garnish)
- 1 tbsp of unsweetened almond yogurt (for garnish)

Directions:
1. Rinse the barley under cold water. In a saucepan, bring the vegetable broth to a boil. Add the barley, reduce the heat to low, cover, and simmer for 25–30 minutes until tender and the liquid is absorbed.
2. Preheat the oven to 375°F. Line a baking sheet with parchment paper.
3. Place the carrots on a baking sheet. Drizzle with olive oil and sprinkle with coriander, turmeric, and salt (if using). Toss to coat evenly. Toss to coat and roast for 20–25 minutes, flipping halfway, until tender and caramelized.
4. In a bowl, combine the cooked barley, roasted carrots, baby spinach, and parsley. Toss gently to mix.
5. Top each serving with a sprinkle of pumpkin seeds. Add a dollop of almond yogurt for a creamy finish.

Shrimp Rice Noodles with Zucchini

 Time:
35 minutes

 Serving Size:
2 servings

 Prep Time:
15 minutes

 Cook Time:
20 minutes

Each Serving Has:
Calories: 292, Carbohydrates: 32g, Saturated Fat: 1g, Protein: 24g, Fat: 9g, Sodium: 170mg, Potassium: 460mg, Fiber: 2g, Sugar: 2g, Vitamin C: 20mg, Calcium: 95mg, Iron: 3mg

Ingredients:
- 6 oz [170g] peeled and deveined medium shrimp
- 1/2 cup [45g] dry thin rice noodles
- 1 cup [130g] thinly sliced zucchini
- 1/4 cup [60ml] unsweetened oat milk
- 1 tsp chopped fresh parsley
- 1/2 tsp chopped fresh dill
- 1 tbsp olive oil

Directions:
1. Bring a medium pot of water to a gentle simmer over medium heat.
2. Add peeled and deveined shrimp and poach for 4–5 minutes, until pink and opaque. Remove shrimp with a slotted spoon and set aside.
3. In the same pot, bring fresh water to a boil. Add dry thin rice noodles and cook for 3–4 minutes, or until tender. Drain and rinse with warm water to prevent sticking.
4. Steam the sliced zucchini in a steamer basket over simmering water for 6–7 minutes, until tender but not mushy. Remove from heat.
5. In a small saucepan over low heat, warm oat milk with chopped parsley, dill, and olive oil. Stir continuously for 2–3 minutes, until herbs are fragrant and sauce is slightly thickened.
6. Arrange cooked rice noodles and steamed zucchini on serving plates. Top with poached shrimp.
7. Drizzle the warm oat milk herb sauce evenly over each plate and serve.

Spinach and Tofu Stir-Fry

 Time:
25 minutes

Serving Size:
2 plates

 Prep Time:
10 minutes

Cook Time:
15 minutes

Each Serving Has:
Calories: 210, Carbohydrates: 12g, Saturated Fat: 1g, Protein: 17g, Fat: 10g, Sodium: 120mg, Potassium: 740mg, Fiber: 4g, Sugar: 4g, Vitamin C: 28mg, Calcium: 150mg, Iron: 4mg.

Ingredients:
- 6 oz [170g] of firm tofu, drained and cubed
- 1 tbsp of olive oil
- 1 cup [30g] of fresh spinach leaves, washed
- 1 medium carrot, julienned
- 1 small zucchini, sliced into half-moons
- 1/4 cup [60ml of] low-sodium vegetable broth
- 1 tbsp of low-sodium soy sauce
- 1 tsp of ground turmeric
- 1 tsp of ground ginger
- 1/2 tsp of sesame seeds (for garnish)

Directions:
1. Heat the olive oil in a large nonstick skillet or wok over medium heat.
2. Add tofu to the skillet and sauté for 5–7 minutes, turning occasionally, until lightly golden on all sides.
3. Push the tofu to one side of the skillet and add the carrot and zucchini. Stir-fry for 3–4 minutes until tender.
4. Add the spinach to the skillet and pour in the vegetable broth and soy sauce. Sprinkle with turmeric and ginger, then stir gently to combine.
5. Continue cooking for 3–4 minutes, allowing the spinach to wilt and the flavors to meld together.
6. Garnish with sesame seeds.

Pumpkin Stew with Barley

Time: 55 minutes	Serving Size: 2 servings
Prep Time: 15 minutes	Cook Time: 40 minutes

Each Serving Has:
Calories: 276, Carbohydrates: 45g, Saturated Fat: 1g, Protein: 8g, Fat: 7g, Sodium: 92mg, Potassium: 835mg, Fiber: 9g, Sugar: 6g, Vitamin C: 24mg, Calcium: 86mg, Iron: 3mg

Ingredients:
- 1/2 cup [100g] hulled barley, rinsed
- 1 3/4 cups [420ml] water
- 1 tsp olive oil
- 1/2 cup [80g] diced peeled pumpkin
- 1/4 cup [30g] chopped celery
- 1/2 cup [120ml] unsweetened oat milk
- 1 cup [30g] chopped fresh spinach
- 1 tbsp chopped fresh parsley

Directions:
1. In a medium saucepan, bring barley and water to a boil. Reduce the heat to low, cover, and simmer for 30–35 minutes, until the barley is tender and most of the liquid has been absorbed. Drain any excess water and set aside.
2. While the barley cooks, heat olive oil in a medium pot over medium-low heat.
3. Sauté diced pumpkin and chopped celery in the olive oil for 8–10 minutes, stirring occasionally, until the vegetables begin to soften.
4. Stir in oat milk and chopped spinach. Reduce heat to low and cover the pot. Simmer gently for 5–7 minutes, until the spinach has wilted and the pumpkin is tender.
5. Add the cooked barley to the pot and stir until well combined. Simmer for an additional 3–4 minutes, allowing the flavors to meld.
6. Stir in chopped parsley. Remove from heat and let sit for 2 minutes.
7. Serve warm.

Broccoli and Sweet Potato Grain Bowl

Time: 30 minutes	Serving Size: 2 bowls
Prep Time: 10 minutes	Cook Time: 20 minutes

Each Serving Has:
Calories: 350, Carbohydrates: 58g, Saturated Fat: 1.5g, Protein: 9g, Fat: 6g, Sodium: 120mg, Potassium: 620mg, Fiber: 9g, Sugar: 7g, Vitamin C: 30mg, Calcium: 70mg, Iron: 2.5mg.

Ingredients:
- 1/2 cup [95g] of quinoa, rinsed
- 1 cup [240ml] of low-sodium vegetable broth
- 1 small sweet potato, peeled and diced (about 1 cup [150g])
- 1 cup [150g] of broccoli florets
- 1 tbsp of olive oil
- 1/2 tsp of ground turmeric
- 1/4 tsp of ground cumin
- 1/8 tsp of ground black pepper
- 1/4 cup[15g] of fresh parsley, chopped (for garnish)
- 1 tbsp of unsalted sunflower seeds (for garnish)

Directions:
1. Cook the quinoa in the broth over medium heat for 15 minutes or until tender. Fluff with a fork and set aside.
2. Preheat the oven to 400°F.
3. Place the sweet potato on a baking sheet, drizzle with 1/2 tbsp of olive oil, and sprinkle with turmeric. Roast in the oven for 15–20 minutes, tossing halfway through, until tender and lightly browned.
4. Steam broccoli for 5–7 minutes until bright green and tender but still crisp.
5. In a bowl, combine the cooked quinoa, roasted sweet potato, and steamed broccoli.
6. Drizzle the remaining olive oil over the mixture, add the cumin and black pepper, and toss until evenly coated.
7. Garnish with parsley and sunflower seeds.

Braised Vegetables with Quinoa

Time:
50 minutes

Serving Size:
2 servings

Prep Time:
15 minutes

Cook Time:
35 minutes

Each Serving Has:
Calories: 298, Carbohydrates: 38g, Saturated Fat: 1g, Protein: 10g, Fat: 12g, Sodium: 78mg, Potassium: 842mg, Fiber: 7g, Sugar: 6g, Vitamin C: 42mg, Calcium: 74mg, Iron: 3mg

Ingredients:
- 1/2 cup [85g] rinsed quinoa
- 1 cup [240ml] water
- 1 tbsp olive oil
- 1/2 cup [70g] diced peeled carrot
- 1/2 cup [80g] chopped zucchini
- 1/2 cup [80g]
- diced peeled sweet potato
- 1/4 cup [60ml] unsweetened almond milk
- 1 tbsp chopped fresh parsley
- 2 tbsp raw pumpkin seeds

Directions:
1. In a small saucepan, bring quinoa and water to a boil. Reduce the heat to low, cover, and simmer for 15–18 minutes, until the quinoa is tender and all the water has been absorbed. Remove from heat and set aside.
2. Meanwhile, heat olive oil in a large skillet over medium-low heat.
3. Sauté diced carrot, chopped zucchini, and sweet potato in the olive oil for 8–10 minutes, stirring occasionally, until the vegetables begin to soften.
4. Pour in almond milk and reduce the heat to low. Cover and simmer for 15 minutes, stirring occasionally, until the vegetables are tender.
5. Stir in the cooked quinoa and continue cooking for 2–3 minutes to allow the mixture to warm through and combine.
6. Sprinkle in chopped parsley, stirring gently to incorporate.
7. Divide the mixture between two bowls and top each serving with raw pumpkin seeds.

Chicken Strips with Wild Rice and Green Beans

Time:
50 minutes

Serving Size:
2 servings

Prep Time:
15 minutes

Cook Time:
35 minutes

Each Serving Has:
Calories: 382, Carbohydrates: 38g, Saturated Fat: 1g, Protein: 33g, Fat: 12g, Sodium: 96mg, Potassium: 742mg, Fiber: 5g, Sugar: 3g, Vitamin C: 19mg, Calcium: 39mg, Iron: 3mg

Ingredients:
- 2/3 cup [125g] rinsed wild rice blend
- 1 1/3 cups [320ml] water
- 1/2 lb [225g] sliced skinless boneless chicken breast
- 1 tbsp olive oil (+ 1 tsp extra for greasing)
- 1/4 tsp dried thyme
- 2 cups [200g] trimmed green beans

Directions:
1. Preheat the oven to 375°F [190°C]. Lightly grease a baking dish with olive oil.
2. In a medium saucepan, bring wild rice blend and water to a boil. Reduce the heat to low, cover, and simmer for 35 minutes, or until the rice is tender and the water is absorbed. Remove from heat and set aside.
3. Arrange sliced chicken breast in the prepared baking dish. Drizzle with olive oil and sprinkle evenly with dried thyme. Toss gently to coat.
4. Bake the chicken in the preheated oven for 25–30 minutes, or until it is fully cooked and no longer pink in the center.
5. While the chicken bakes, steam the trimmed green beans in a steamer basket over boiling water for 8–10 minutes, until they are bright green and tender.
6. Divide the cooked wild rice between two plates. Top with baked chicken strips and steamed green beans. Serve warm.

Creamy Broccoli and Rice Soup

Time: 30 minutes	Serving Size: 2 bowls
Prep Time: 10 minutes	Cook Time: 20 minutes

Each Serving Has:
Calories: 200, Carbohydrates: 32g, Saturated Fat: 1.5g, Protein: 6g, Fat: 5g, Sodium: 140mg, Potassium: 450mg, Fiber: 4g, Sugar: 3g, Vitamin C: 40mg, Calcium: 80mg, Iron: 2mg.

Ingredients:
- 1 cup [240ml] of low-sodium vegetable broth
- 1 cup [240ml] of unsweetened almond milk
- 1/2 cup [100g] of cooked brown rice
- 1 1/2 cups [150g] of broccoli florets, chopped into small pieces
- 1/2 medium carrot, diced
- 1/2 medium zucchini, diced
- 1/4 medium onion, finely chopped
- 1 tbsp of olive oil
- 1/4 tsp of ground turmeric
- 1/4 tsp of ground cumin

Directions:
1. Heat olive oil in a medium-sized pot over medium heat. Add onion and sauté for 2-3 minutes until softened.
2. Stir in carrot and zucchini. Cook for another 3-4 minutes, stirring occasionally.
3. Add the broccoli florets, turmeric, and cumin to the pot. Stir to coat the vegetables with the spices.
4. Pour in the vegetable broth, bring to a boil, then reduce the heat to low, cover, and simmer for 10 minutes until the vegetables are tender.
5. Add the almond milk and cooked brown rice to the pot. Simmer for 5 minutes.
6. Use an immersion blender to puree part of the soup in the pot, leaving some pieces for texture. Alternatively, blend half and return it to the pot.
7. Stir the soup well, adjust the seasoning if needed.

Butternut Squash and Quinoa Pilaf with Dill

Time: 30 minutes	Serving Size: 2 bowls
Prep Time: 10 minutes	Cook Time: 20 minutes

Each Serving Has:
Calories: 285, Carbohydrates: 45g, Saturated Fat: 1g, Protein: 7g, Fat: 8g, Sodium: 70mg, Potassium: 590mg, Fiber: 5g, Sugar: 4g, Vitamin C: 15mg, Calcium: 40mg, Iron: 2mg

Ingredients:
- 1/2 cup [95g] uncooked quinoa
- 1 cup [240ml] low-sodium vegetable broth
- 1 cup [150g] diced butternut squash
- 1/4 cup [35g] finely chopped yellow onion
- 1 tbsp olive oil
- 1 tbsp fresh dill, chopped
- 1/4 tsp ground coriander
- 1/4 tsp ground cumin
- 1/4 tsp sea salt (optional)
- 1/4 tsp ground turmeric

Directions:
1. Rinse the quinoa under cold water until the water runs clear.
2. In a saucepan, heat the olive oil over medium heat. Add onion and sauté for 2–3 minutes until softened.
3. Add the butternut squash to the pan and cook for an additional 5 minutes, stirring occasionally.
4. Stir in the quinoa, coriander, cumin, turmeric, and sea salt (if using). Mix well to coat the quinoa and butternut squash in the spices.
5. Pour in the vegetable broth, bring to a boil, then reduce the heat to low. Cover and simmer for 15 minutes, or until the quinoa absorbs the liquid and the butternut squash is tender.
6. Remove the saucepan from the heat and let it sit, covered, for 5 minutes. Fluff the quinoa with a fork.
7. Stir in dill, mixing gently to combine the flavors.

Roasted Pumpkin and Fennel Bowl

 Time: 40 minutes	Serving Size: 2 bowls
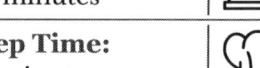 Prep Time: 10 minutes	Cook Time: 30 minutes

Each Serving Has:

Calories: 280, Carbohydrates: 45g, Saturated Fat: 1g, Protein: 6g, Fat: 8g, Sodium: 120mg, Potassium: 540mg, Fiber: 7g, Sugar: 6g, Vitamin C: 45mg, Calcium: 60mg, Iron: 2mg.

Ingredients:

- 2 cups [400g] of cubed pumpkin
- 1 small fennel bulb, thinly sliced
- 1 cup [200g] of cooked quinoa
- 1 tbsp of olive oil
- 1/2 tsp of ground turmeric
- 1/2 tsp of ground cumin
- 1/4 tsp of ground cinnamon
- 1/8 tsp of sea salt
- 1/4 cup [60ml] of plain unsweetened coconut yogurt (for garnish)
- 1 tbsp of fresh parsley, chopped (for garnish)

Directions:

1. Preheat the oven to 375°F. Line a baking sheet with parchment paper.
2. Place the pumpkin and fennel on the prepared baking sheet. Drizzle with olive oil and sprinkle with turmeric, cumin, cinnamon, and sea salt. Toss until evenly coated.
3. Roast the vegetables in the preheated oven for 25-30 minutes, stirring halfway through, until the pumpkin is tender and the fennel is lightly caramelized.
4. While the vegetables are roasting, warm the cooked quinoa in a small saucepan over low heat or in the microwave.
5. Divide the warmed quinoa between two bowls. Top with the roasted pumpkin and fennel.
6. Add a dollop of coconut yogurt to each bowl and garnish with chopped parsley.

Baked Bell Peppers with Quinoa

Time: 50 minutes	Serving Size: 2 servings
Prep Time: 20 minutes	Cook Time: 30 minutes

Each Serving Has:

Calories: 232, Carbohydrates: 34g, Saturated Fat: 1g, Protein: 7g, Fat: 7g, Sodium: 58mg, Potassium: 520mg, Fiber: 5g, Sugar: 5g, Vitamin C: 135mg, Calcium: 35mg, Iron: 2mg

Ingredients:

- 1/2 cup [85g] rinsed quinoa
- 1 cup [240ml] water
- 2 medium orange or yellow bell peppers, halved lengthwise and seeded
- 1/2 cup [45g]
- grated carrot
- 1/2 cup [30g] chopped fresh spinach leaves
- 1 tbsp chopped fresh parsley
- 3 tsp olive oil
- 1/4 tsp dried thyme

Directions:

1. Preheat the oven to 375°F [190°C].
2. In a small saucepan, bring quinoa and water to a boil over medium heat. Add quinoa, reduce heat to low, cover, and simmer 15 minutes until tender and liquid is absorbed. Remove from heat and let sit, covered.
3. Lightly brush the halved bell peppers with 1 teaspoon of olive oil and place them cut-side up in a baking dish.
4. In a small nonstick pan, sauté grated carrot in 2 teaspoons of olive oil over low heat for 3 minutes, until softened. Add chopped spinach and cook 2 more minutes until wilted. Remove from heat.
5. In a bowl, combine the cooked quinoa, sautéed vegetables, chopped parsley, and dried thyme. Mix well.
6. Spoon the mixture into the bell pepper halves, pressing gently to compact the filling.
7. Cover the baking dish with foil and bake for 25 minutes. Remove the foil and bake for another 5 minutes, until the tops are golden and the peppers are tender.
8. Let cool slightly before serving.

Steamed Halibut with Dill Rice and Tender Chayote

Time: 25 minutes	Serving Size: 2 plates
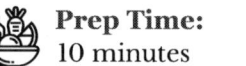 Prep Time: 10 minutes	Cook Time: 15 minutes

Each Serving Has:
Calories: 360, Carbohydrates: 46g, Saturated Fat: 1g, Protein: 29g, Fat: 7g, Sodium: 210mg, Potassium: 740mg, Fiber: 5g, Sugar: 2g, Vitamin C: 16mg, Calcium: 50mg, Iron: 2mg

Ingredients:
- 2 halibut fillets (6 oz [170g] each)
- 1 cup [180g] long-grain brown rice
- 2 cups [480ml] water
- 1 tbsp olive oil
- 1 tbsp fresh dill, finely chopped
- 1 small chayote squash (5 oz [150g]), peeled and diced
- 1 small kohlrabi (5 oz [150g]), peeled and thinly sliced
- 1/4 tsp sea salt

Directions:
1. Rinse the brown rice until the water runs clear. Boil water in a saucepan, then add rice and a pinch of salt. Reduce heat and simmer covered on low for about 45 minutes, or until tender and the water is absorbed.
2. Place the chopped chayote and sliced kohlrabi in a steamer basket over a pot of gently simmering water. Cover and steam for 8–10 minutes or until tender. Remove and set aside.
3. Season the halibut fillets with the remaining sea salt. Place them in the steamer basket over fresh simmering water. Cover and steam for 10–12 minutes or until the fish is flaky.
4. Once the rice is cooked, remove it from heat and fluff with a fork. Stir in the olive oil and chopped dill. Stir in steamed chayote and kohlrabi.
5. Divide the rice and vegetables between two plates and top each with a halibut fillet.

Cauliflower and Zucchini Casserole

Time: 45 minutes	Serving Size: 2 bowls
Prep Time: 15 minutes	Cook Time: 30 minutes

Each Serving Has:
Calories: 220, Carbohydrates: 22g, Saturated Fat: 1g, Protein: 6g, Fat: 12g, Sodium: 150mg, Potassium: 650mg, Fiber: 6g, Sugar: 7g, Vitamin C: 65mg, Calcium: 120mg, Iron: 1.5mg.

Ingredients:
- 1 small cauliflower head (about 1 lb [453.6g])
- 1 medium zucchini (about 6 oz [170g]), sliced
- 1/2 cup [120ml] of unsweetened almond milk
- 1 tbsp of olive oil
- 1/4 cup [30g] of shredded reduced-fat Parmesan cheese
- 1/2 tsp of garlic powder
- 1/2 tsp of dried oregano
- 1/8 tsp of sea salt
- 1/2 cup [50g] of panko breadcrumbs (optional)

Directions:
1. Preheat the oven to 375°F [190°C].
2. Steam or microwave the cauliflower for about 8-10 minutes until tender.
3. While the cauliflower is cooking, heat olive oil in a large skillet over medium heat. Add the zucchini slices and sauté for 5-6 minutes until slightly softened. Remove from heat and set aside.
4. In a mixing bowl, combine the steamed cauliflower, sautéed zucchini, almond milk, Parmesan, garlic powder, oregano, and sea salt. Stir well to combine all ingredients.
5. Transfer the mixture to a greased baking dish (about 8x8 inches [20x20 cm]). If desired, top with panko breadcrumbs.
6. Bake in the preheated oven for 20-25 minutes, or until the casserole is golden on top and bubbly.
7. Garnish with extra Parmesan cheese if preferred.

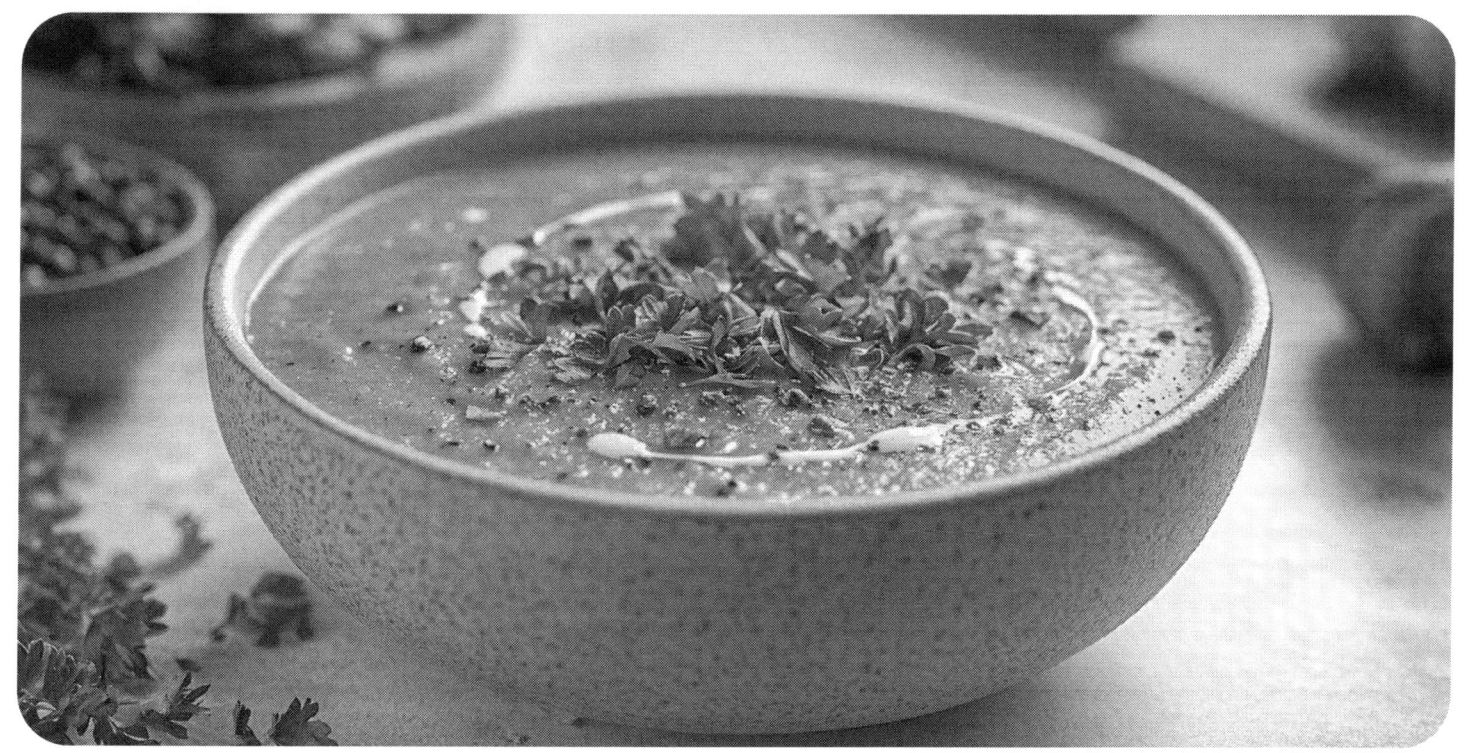

Chapter 5: Salads and Soups

Millet and Roasted Zucchini Salad with Dill

Time: 45 minutes	**Serving Size:** 2 servings
Prep Time: 15 minutes	**Cook Time:** 30 minutes

Each Serving Has:
Calories: 292, Carbohydrates: 38g, Saturated Fat: 1g, Protein: 7g, Fat: 12g, Sodium: 22mg, Potassium: 488mg, Fiber: 5g, Sugar: 4g, Vitamin C: 29mg, Calcium: 36mg, Iron: 2mg

Ingredients:
- 1/2 cup [90g] rinsed millet
- 1 1/2 cups [360ml] water
- 1 1/2 cups [180g] chopped zucchini
- 1 tbsp olive oil
- 1/2 cup [60g] diced peeled cucumber
- 1/4 cup [10g] chopped fresh parsley
- 1 tbsp chopped fresh dill
- 1 tbsp freshly squeezed pear juice

Directions:
1. Preheat the oven to 375°F [190°C]. Line a baking tray with parchment paper.

2. In a medium saucepan, bring millet and water to a boil. Reduce the heat to low, cover, and simmer for 20 minutes, or until the water is absorbed and the millet is tender. Remove from heat and let it sit, covered, for 5 minutes.

3. While the millet cooks, spread chopped zucchini on the prepared baking tray. Drizzle with olive oil and toss to coat evenly.

4. Roast the zucchini in a preheated oven for 20 minutes, stirring once halfway through, until it is lightly golden and tender. Remove from the oven and set aside to cool slightly.

5. In a large bowl, combine cooked millet, roasted zucchini, diced cucumber, chopped parsley, and dill.

6. Drizzle with pear juice and toss gently to blend the flavors.

7. Let the salad sit for 5 minutes before serving.

Quinoa and Cucumber Salad with Fresh Dill

 Time:
20 minutes

 Serving Size:
2 bowls

 Prep Time:
10 minutes

 Cook Time:
10 minutes

Each Serving Has:
Calories: 180, Carbohydrates: 32g, Saturated Fat: 0g, Protein: 5g, Fat: 6g, Sodium: 30mg, Potassium: 380mg, Fiber: 4g, Sugar: 3g, Vitamin C: 6mg, Calcium: 30mg, Iron: 1.5mg.

Ingredients:
- 1/2 cup [90g] of quinoa
- 1 cup [200g] of cucumber, peeled and diced
- 1 tbsp [15ml] of olive oil
- 1 tbsp [15ml] of
- lemon juice
- 1 tbsp [15g] of fresh dill, chopped
- 1 tbsp [15g] of fresh parsley, chopped
- 1/6 of tsp salt

Directions:
1. Rinse the quinoa under cold water. In a medium pot, bring 1 cup [240ml] of water to a boil. Add the quinoa, reduce the heat, and cover the pot. Simmer for about 10 minutes, or until the quinoa is cooked and the water is absorbed. Remove from heat and let it cool slightly.
2. While the quinoa is cooking, prepare the cucumber and chop the fresh dill and parsley.
3. Once the quinoa has cooled, fluff it with a fork and transfer it to a mixing bowl.
4. Add cucumber, dill, and parsley to the quinoa.
5. Drizzle the olive oil and lemon juice over the salad, and sprinkle with salt. Toss everything together gently until well combined.

Carrot, Fennel, and Quinoa Warm Salad

 Time:
40 minutes

 Serving Size:
2 servings

 Prep Time:
15 minutes

Cook Time:
25 minutes

Each Serving Has:
Calories: 278, Carbohydrates: 39g, Saturated Fat: 1g, Protein: 7g, Fat: 10g, Sodium: 40mg, Potassium: 656mg, Fiber: 6g, Sugar: 7g, Vitamin C: 19mg, Calcium: 65mg, Iron: 2mg

Ingredients:
- 1/2 cup [85g] rinsed quinoa
- 1 1/4 cups [300ml] water
- 1/2 cup [60g] thinly sliced fennel bulb
- 3/4 cup [90g] peeled and thinly
- sliced carrots
- 1 tbsp olive oil
- 1 tbsp chopped fresh parsley
- 1 tbsp chopped fresh dill
- 2 tbsp unsweetened pear juice

Directions:
1. In a medium saucepan, combine quinoa and water. Bring to a boil over medium-high heat, then reduce the heat to low, cover, and simmer for 15 minutes, or until the water is absorbed and the quinoa is tender. Remove from heat and let it sit, covered, for 5 minutes.
2. While the quinoa cooks, heat olive oil in a nonstick skillet over medium heat.
3. Add thinly sliced fennel and carrots to the skillet. Sauté gently for 8–10 minutes, stirring occasionally, until the vegetables are soft and lightly golden.
4. In a large bowl, combine cooked quinoa, sautéed fennel and carrots, chopped parsley, and dill.
5. Drizzle the mixture with pear juice and toss gently to coat.
6. Serve the warm salad immediately.

Green Bean and Buckwheat Salad

 Time: 35 minutes

 Serving Size: 2 servings

 Prep Time: 10 minutes

Cook Time: 25 minutes

Each Serving Has:
Calories: 278, Carbohydrates: 37g, Saturated Fat: 1g, Protein: 9g, Fat: 10g, Sodium: 18mg, Potassium: 504mg, Fiber: 6g, Sugar: 4g, Vitamin C: 22mg, Calcium: 52mg, Iron: 2mg

Ingredients:
- 1/2 cup [85g] rinsed buckwheat groats
- 1 cup [240ml] water
- 1 1/2 cups [150g] trimmed and halved green beans
- 1/4 cup [30g]
- grated carrot
- 2 tbsp raw pumpkin seeds
- 1 tbsp chopped fresh dill
- 1 tbsp chopped fresh parsley
- 1 tbsp olive oil
- 2 tbsp lime juice

Directions:
1. In a medium saucepan, combine buckwheat groats and water. Bring to a boil over medium-high heat, then reduce the heat to low, cover, and simmer for 15 minutes, or until the buckwheat is tender and the water is absorbed. Remove from heat and let stand covered for 5 minutes.
2. While the buckwheat cooks, place halved green beans in a steamer basket over simmering water. Cover and steam for 6–8 minutes until just tender. Remove from heat and set aside.
3. In a dry skillet over medium-low heat, lightly toast raw pumpkin seeds for 2–3 minutes, stirring frequently until fragrant. Remove from heat.
4. In a large bowl, combine cooked buckwheat, steamed green beans, grated carrot, chopped dill, parsley, and toasted pumpkin seeds.
5. Drizzle the mixture with olive oil and lime juice. Toss gently to coat all ingredients evenly.
6. Serve warm.

Chilled Cucumber and Yogurt Soup

 Time: 15 minutes

 Serving Size: 2 bowls

 Prep Time: 15 minutes

Cook Time: 0 minutes

Each Serving Has:
Calories: 120, Carbohydrates: 12g, Saturated Fat: 2g, Protein: 6g, Fat: 8g, Sodium: 60mg, Potassium: 350mg, Fiber: 2g, Sugar: 5g, Vitamin C: 10mg, Calcium: 90mg, Iron: 0.5mg.

Ingredients:
- 1 medium cucumber, peeled and chopped
- 1 cup [240g] of plain Greek yogurt
- 1/4 cup [10g] of fresh dill, chopped
- 1 tbsp of olive oil
- [15ml]
- 1/8 tsp of ground white pepper
- 1/8 tsp of salt
- 1/4 cup [60ml] of water
- Ice cubes (optional)

Directions:
1. In a blender or food processor, combine the cucumber, Greek yogurt, dill, olive oil, white pepper, and salt.
2. Add 1/4 cup of water and blend until smooth and creamy. If you prefer a thinner consistency, add additional water, 1 tbsp at a time.
3. Chill the soup in the refrigerator for at least 10 minutes to allow the flavors to meld together. Alternatively, you can add ice cubes directly into the soup before serving for extra coolness.
4. Once chilled, serve the soup garnished with additional fresh dill, if desired.

Creamy Lentil and Spinach Soup

 Time: 30 minutes

 Serving Size: 2 bowls

 Prep Time: 10 minutes

 Cook Time: 20 minutes

Each Serving Has:
Calories: 220, Carbohydrates: 35g, Saturated Fat: 2g, Protein: 12g, Fat: 6g, Sodium: 150mg, Potassium: 550mg, Fiber: 10g, Sugar: 4g, Vitamin C: 10mg, Calcium: 80mg, Iron: 2.5mg.

Ingredients:
- 1/2 cup [90g] of dry green lentils
- 2 cups [480ml] of vegetable broth
- 2 cups [60g] of fresh spinach, chopped
- 1 small of onion, chopped
- 1 tbsp [15ml] of olive oil
- 1/2 tsp of ground cumin
- 1/4 tsp of ground turmeric
- 1/2 cup [120ml] of unsweetened almond milk
- 1/8 tsp of salt
- 1 tbsp of fresh parsley, chopped (for garnish)

Directions:
1. Rinse the lentils under cold water and set aside.
2. Heat the olive oil in a medium pot over medium heat. Add the onion and sauté for 3-4 minutes until softened and fragrant.
3. Add cumin, turmeric and salt to the onions, stirring to combine. Let the spices cook for 1 minute to release their aromas.
4. Stir in the lentils and vegetable broth. Bring the mixture to a boil, then reduce the heat to low and simmer for 15-20 minutes, or until the lentils are tender.
5. Add spinach to the pot and stir it in. Let it wilt in the hot soup for about 2 minutes.
6. Stir in the almond milk, and allow the soup to heat through for another 2-3 minutes.
7. Garnish with fresh parsley.

Low-Acid Pumpkin Soup with Parsley

 Time: 30 minutes

 Serving Size: 2 bowls

 Prep Time: 10 minutes

 Cook Time: 20 minutes

Each Serving Has:
Calories: 180, Carbohydrates: 35g, Saturated Fat: 1g, Protein: 4g, Fat: 4g, Sodium: 300mg, Potassium: 700mg, Fiber: 7g, Sugar: 8g, Vitamin C: 15mg, Calcium: 60mg, Iron: 2mg.

Ingredients:
- 2 cups [480g] of pumpkin puree
- 1 small onion, diced
- 1 tbsp [15ml] of olive oil
- 2 cups [480ml] of vegetable broth
- 1/2 tsp of ground ginger
- 1/4 tsp ground nutmeg
- 1/4 tsp of ground cinnamon
- 1 tbsp of fresh parsley, chopped (for garnish)
- 1/2 cup [120ml] of unsweetened almond milk
- 1/8 tsp of salt

Directions:
1. Heat olive oil in a medium pot over medium heat. Add onion and sauté for 3-4 minutes, until softened and translucent.
2. Add the pumpkin puree to the pot, stirring to combine with the onion. Let it cook for 2-3 minutes to release its natural sweetness.
3. Pour in the vegetable broth and stir in ginger, nutmeg, cinnamon, and salt. Bring the mixture to a gentle simmer and cook for 10-12 minutes, stirring occasionally.
4. Once the soup is heated through and the flavors are well combined, add the almond milk. Stir to combine and let the soup cook for an additional 2-3 minutes.
5. Use an immersion blender to blend the soup until smooth, or transfer the mixture in batches to a blender.
6. Ladle the soup into bowls and garnish with fresh chopped parsley. Serve warm.

Millet and Herb Vegetable Soup

 Time:
35 minutes

 Serving Size:
2 bowls

Prep Time:
10 minutes

Cook Time:
25 minutes

Each Serving Has:
Calories: 220, Carbohydrates: 46g, Saturated Fat: 1g, Protein: 6g, Fat: 3g, Sodium: 320mg, Potassium: 700mg, Fiber: 8g, Sugar: 5g, Vitamin C: 30mg, Calcium: 60mg, Iron: 3mg.

Ingredients:
- 1/2 cup [90g] of millet
- 2 cups [480ml] of vegetable broth
- 1 medium zucchini, diced
- 1 medium carrot, peeled and diced
- 1/2 cup [70g] of celery, diced
- 1/2 cup [15g] of
- spinach, fresh
- 1/4 cup [15g] of fresh parsley, chopped
- 1/4 tsp of dried thyme
- 1/4 tsp of dried oregano
- 1 tbsp [15g] of olive oil
- 1/8 tsp of salt

Directions:
1. Begin by rinsing the millet under cold water in a fine-mesh sieve.
2. In a medium pot, heat the olive oil over medium heat. Add the diced carrots, zucchini, and celery. Sauté the vegetables for 5 minutes, stirring occasionally, until they begin to soften.
3. Add the vegetable broth to the pot, followed by the rinsed millet. Stir in the thyme, oregano, and salt. Bring the mixture to a boil.
4. Once boiling, reduce the heat to low, cover, and let the soup simmer for 15-20 minutes, or until the millet is tender and has absorbed most of the liquid.
5. Stir in spinach and parsley, cooking for an additional 2-3 minutes until the spinach wilts.
6. Serve the soup warm, garnished with extra fresh parsley, if desired.

Roasted Cauliflower and Broccoli Soup

 Time:
45 minutes

 Serving Size:
2 bowls

Prep Time:
10 minutes

Cook Time:
35 minutes

Each Serving Has:
Calories: 210, Carbohydrates: 34g, Saturated Fat: 2g, Protein: 6g, Fat: 7g, Sodium: 320mg, Potassium: 710mg, Fiber: 10g, Sugar: 7g, Vitamin C: 85mg, Calcium: 60mg, Iron: 2mg.

Ingredients:
- 1 small cauliflower, cut into florets
- 1 small head of broccoli, cut into florets
- 1 tbsp [15g] of olive oil
- 1/2 medium onion, diced
- 2 cups [480ml] of vegetable broth
- 1/2 tsp of dried thyme
- 1/8 tsp of salt
- 1/4 cup [60ml] of unsweetened almond milk
- fresh herbs (optional)

Directions:
1. Preheat the oven to 400°F [200°C].
2. Toss the cauliflower and broccoli with 1 tbsp of olive oil on a baking sheet. Roast in the oven for 20-25 minutes, stirring halfway through, until tender.
3. Heat a small amount of olive oil in a pot over medium heat. Add the diced onion and cook for 3-4 minutes, until soft.
4. Once the cauliflower and broccoli are roasted, add them to the pot with the onion. Stir in the vegetable broth and thyme. Bring to a simmer and cook for 10 more minutes to blend the flavors.
5. Use an immersion blender to puree the soup until creamy, or transfer it to a blender and blend in batches.
6. Once blended, return the soup to the heat, stir in the almond milk, and season with salt. Heat through.
7. Optionally garnish with a sprinkle of fresh herbs.

Steamed Carrot and Wild Rice Salad

🕐 **Time:** 35 minutes	🍽 **Serving Size:** 2 plates
🥗 **Prep Time:** 10 minutes	👨‍🍳 **Cook Time:** 25 minutes

Each Serving Has:
Calories: 230, Carbohydrates: 48g, Saturated Fat: 1g, Protein: 6g, Fat: 3g, Sodium: 30mg, Potassium: 500mg, Fiber: 7g, Sugar: 9g, Vitamin C: 25mg, Calcium: 40mg, Iron: 2mg.

Ingredients:
- 1/2 cup [90g] of wild rice
- 2 medium carrots, peeled and sliced
- 1 tbsp [15ml] of olive oil
- 1 tbsp [15ml] of fresh lemon juice
- 1/2 tsp of dried oregano
- 1/8 tsp of salt
- 2 tbsp of fresh parsley, chopped (for garnish)

Directions:

1. Rinse the wild rice under cold water. In a medium saucepan, add the rice and 1 cup [240ml] of water. Bring to a boil, then reduce the heat to low, cover, and simmer for about 25 minutes, or until tender and the water is absorbed.
2. While the rice is cooking, steam the carrots. Place carrots in a steamer basket over boiling water. Cover and steam for about 8-10 minutes, or until they are tender but still vibrant.
3. Once the rice is cooked, fluff it with a fork and transfer it to a large bowl. Add the steamed carrots.
4. Drizzle the olive oil and lemon juice over the rice and carrots. Sprinkle with oregano, and salt. Stir everything gently to combine and coat evenly.
5. Garnish the salad with chopped fresh parsley.

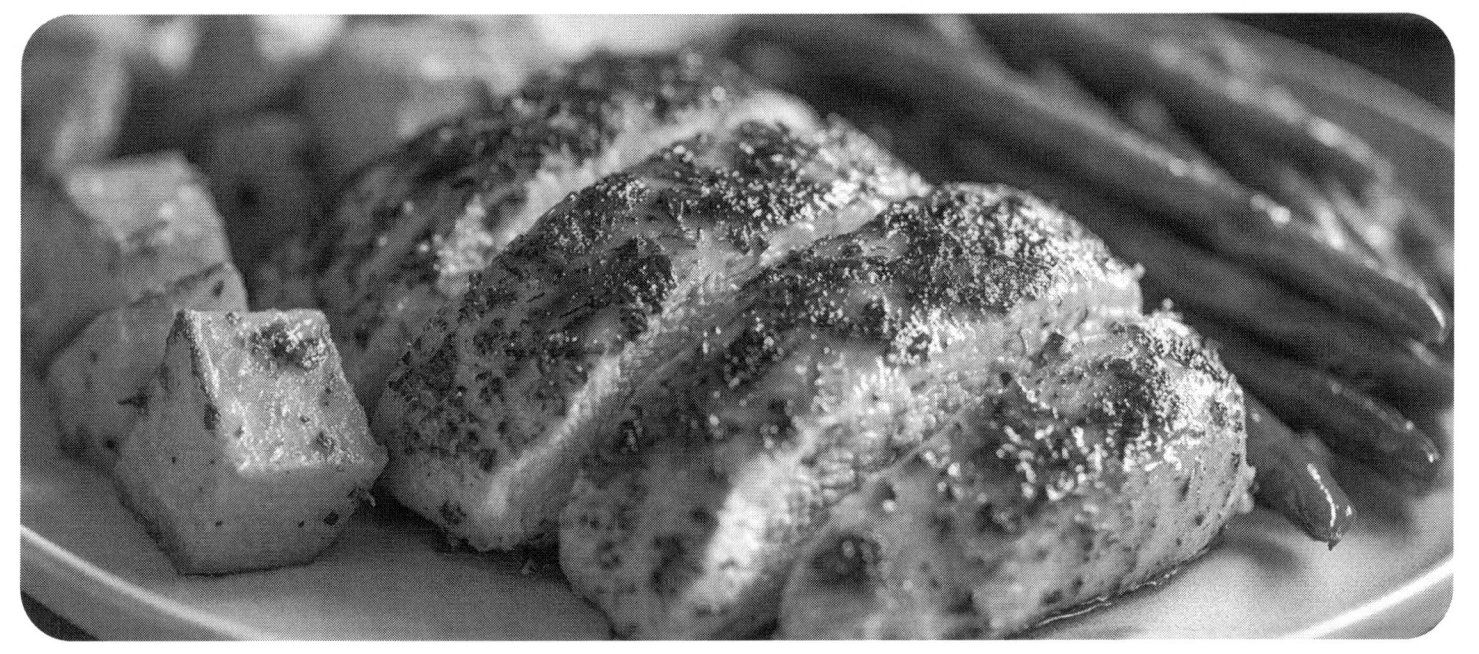

Chapter 6: Dinner

Chicken Thighs with Barley and Carrots

Time: 55 minutes	Serving Size: 2 servings
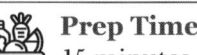 Prep Time: 15 minutes	Cook Time: 40 minutes

Each Serving Has:
Calories: 384, Carbohydrates: 34g, Saturated Fat: 2g, Protein: 30g, Fat: 15g, Sodium: 102mg, Potassium: 610mg, Fiber: 5g, Sugar: 4g, Vitamin C: 7mg, Calcium: 37mg, Iron: 3mg

Ingredients:
- 2 skinless boneless chicken thighs [200g]
- 1/2 cup [90g] rinsed pearl barley
- 1 1/2 cups [360ml] water
- 1 cup [120g] peeled and diagonally sliced carrots
- 1 tbsp chopped fresh parsley
- 1/2 tsp dried thyme
- 1/4 tsp sea salt (optional)
- 1 tbsp olive oil

Directions:
1. Preheat the oven to 375°F [190°C]. Lightly grease a small baking dish with a bit of olive oil.
2. Arrange chicken thighs in the prepared baking dish. Drizzle with olive oil, then sprinkle with chopped parsley, dried thyme, and sea salt (if using).
3. Cover the dish with foil and bake for 30 minutes. Uncover and bake for an additional 10 minutes, or until the chicken is cooked through and tender.
4. While the chicken bakes, combine rinsed pearl barley and water in a medium saucepan. Bring to a boil over medium-high heat, then reduce the heat to low, cover, and simmer for 30–35 minutes, or until the barley is tender and the liquid has been absorbed. Remove from heat and let stand, covered, for 5 minutes.
5. While the barley simmers, place the sliced carrots in a steamer basket over simmering water. Cover and steam for 8–10 minutes until fork-tender. Remove from heat.
6. To serve, divide the cooked barley and steamed carrots between two plates and top each with a baked chicken thigh. Spoon any remaining pan juices from the baking dish over the chicken.

Millet and Spinach Bake with Dill Sauce

Time: 55 minutes	Serving Size: 2 servings
Prep Time: 20 minutes	Cook Time: 35 minutes

Each Serving Has:
Calories: 336, Carbohydrates: 42g, Saturated Fat: 1g, Protein: 11g, Fat: 13g, Sodium: 96mg, Potassium: 532mg, Fiber: 5g, Sugar: 3g, Vitamin C: 16mg, Calcium: 97mg, Iron: 3mg

Ingredients:
- 1/2 cup [85g] rinsed millet
- 1 1/4 cups [300ml] water
- 1 cup [60g] chopped fresh spinach
- 1 tbsp chopped fresh dill
- 1/2 cup [120ml] unsweetened oat
- milk
- 1 tbsp oat flour
- 1 tbsp nutritional yeast
- 1 tbsp olive oil (+ 1/2 tsp extra for greasing)
- 1/8 tsp ground white pepper (optional)

Directions:
1. Preheat the oven to 375°F [190°C]. Line a baking tray with parchment paper.
2. In a medium saucepan, bring millet and water to a boil. Reduce the heat to low, cover, and simmer for 20 minutes, or until the water is absorbed and the millet is tender. Remove from heat and let it sit, covered, for 5 minutes.
3. While the millet cooks, spread chopped zucchini on the prepared baking tray. Drizzle with olive oil and toss to coat evenly.
4. Roast the zucchini in a preheated oven for 20 minutes, stirring once halfway through, until it is lightly golden and tender. Remove from the oven and set aside to cool slightly.
5. In a large bowl, combine cooked millet, roasted zucchini, diced cucumber, chopped parsley, and dill.
6. Drizzle with pear juice and toss gently to blend the flavors.
7. Let the salad sit for 5 minutes before serving.

White Fish with Zucchini and Quinoa

Time: 35 minutes	Serving Size: 2 servings
Prep Time: 15 minutes	Cook Time: 20 minutes

Each Serving Has:
Calories: 321, Carbohydrates: 28g, Saturated Fat: 1g, Protein: 30g, Fat: 11g, Sodium: 82mg, Potassium: 706mg, Fiber: 4g, Sugar: 3g, Vitamin C: 21mg, Calcium: 46mg, Iron: 3mg

Ingredients:
- 2 fillets [300g] skinless white fish (e.g., cod or haddock)
- 1 1/2 cups [360ml] low-sodium vegetable broth
- 1/2 cup [85g] rinsed quinoa
- 1 cup [240ml] water
- 1 cup [120g] thinly sliced zucchini ribbons
- 1 tbsp chopped fresh parsley
- 1 tbsp olive oil
- 1/8 tsp sea salt
- 1/4 tsp ground white pepper (optional)

Directions:
1. Boil water in a small saucepan. Stir in rinsed quinoa, cover, and simmer 15 minutes until tender and water is absorbed. Remove from heat and keep covered.
2. Pour the vegetable broth into a wide skillet and bring to a gentle simmer over medium heat.
3. Carefully place the white fish fillets into the simmering broth. Cover and poach for 8–10 minutes, or until the fish is opaque and flaky. Remove from the broth and keep warm.
4. Heat olive oil in a skillet over medium heat. Sauté zucchini ribbons 2–3 minutes until tender but not mushy.
5. In a large bowl, combine the cooked quinoa, sautéed zucchini ribbons, chopped parsley, sea salt, and white pepper (if using). Toss gently to mix.
6. Divide the quinoa and zucchini mixture between two plates. Top each serving with a poached fish fillet and serve.

Quinoa and Roasted Pumpkin Bowl

 Time: 40 minutes

 Prep Time: 15 minutes

Serving Size: 2 bowls

Cook Time: 25 minutes

Each Serving Has:
Calories: 320, Carbohydrates: 58g, Saturated Fat: 2g, Protein: 8g, Fat: 7g, Sodium: 12mg, Potassium: 630mg, Fiber: 8g, Sugar: 10g, Vitamin C: 15mg, Calcium: 50mg, Iron: 2mg.

Ingredients:
- 1/2 cup [90g] of quinoa
- 1 small pumpkin (about 2 cups cubed) [240g]
- 1 tbsp [15ml] of olive oil
- 1/2 tsp of ground cinnamon
- 1/2 tsp of ground ginger
- 1/8 tsp of salt
- 1 tbsp of fresh parsley, chopped (for garnish)
- 1 tbsp [15ml] of tahini
- 2 tbsp [30ml] of water
- 1 tsp of lemon zest

Directions:
1. Preheat the oven to 400°F [200°C].
2. Toss the pumpkin with 1 tbsp olive oil, cinnamon, ginger, and salt. Arrange the pumpkin cubes on a baking sheet in a single layer. Roast in the oven for 25 minutes, or until tender and lightly browned, flipping halfway through.
3. While the pumpkin is roasting, rinse the quinoa under cold water. In a saucepan, combine the quinoa and 1 cup of water [240ml]. Bring to a boil, then reduce to a simmer. Cover and cook for 12-15 minutes, or until the quinoa is fluffy and the water is absorbed.
4. In a bowl, whisk together tahini, 2 tbsp water [30ml], and lemon zest until smooth. Adjust the consistency with additional water if needed.
5. Once the pumpkin and quinoa are ready, top with the roasted pumpkin cubes and drizzle with the tahini dressing.
6. Garnish with freshly chopped parsley.

Barley Pilaf with Roasted Carrots

 Time: 45 minutes

  Prep Time: 15 minutes

 Serving Size: 2 plates

Cook Time: 30 minutes

Each Serving Has:
Calories: 270, Carbohydrates: 58g, Saturated Fat: 1g, Protein: 6g, Fat: 4g, Sodium: 25mg, Potassium: 650mg, Fiber: 8g, Sugar: 8g, Vitamin C: 9mg, Calcium: 35mg, Iron: 2mg.

Ingredients:
- 1/2 cup [90g] of barley
- 2 medium carrots, peeled and cut into 1/2-inch [1.25cm] pieces
- 1 tbsp [15ml] of olive oil
- 1/2 tsp of ground turmeric
- 1/2 tsp of ground cumin
- 1/8 tsp of salt
- 2 cups [480ml] of vegetable broth
- 1 tbsp of fresh parsley, chopped
- 1 tbsp [15ml] of lemon juice

Directions:
1. Preheat the oven to 400°F [200°C].
2. Place the carrot pieces on a baking sheet, drizzle with 1 tbsp olive oil, and sprinkle with turmeric, cumin, and salt. Toss to coat evenly. Roast in the oven for 20-25 minutes, flipping halfway through, until tender and lightly browned.
3. While the carrots are roasting, rinse the barley under cold water. In a saucepan, bring 2 cups vegetable broth [480ml] to a boil. Add the barley and a pinch of salt. Reduce the heat to low, cover, and simmer for 25-30 minutes, or until the barley is tender and the liquid is absorbed.
4. Once the barley and roasted carrots are ready, fluff the barley with a fork.
5. In a bowl, combine the cooked barley with the roasted carrots. Stir in the fresh parsley and lemon juice.

Fish Fillets with Steamed Green Beans

Time: 30 minutes	Serving Size: 2 plates
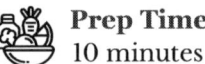 Prep Time: 10 minutes	Cook Time: 20 minutes

Each Serving Has:

Calories: 280, Carbohydrates: 18g, Saturated Fat: 1g, Protein: 26g, Fat: 12g, Sodium: 120mg, Potassium: 800mg, Fiber: 5g, Sugar: 4g, Vitamin C: 18mg, Calcium: 70mg, Iron: 2mg.

Ingredients:

- 2 white fish fillets (such as cod or tilapia) [6 oz (170g) each]
- 1 tbsp [15ml] of olive oil
- 1 tsp of dried oregano
- 1 tsp of dried thyme
- 1/8 tsp of salt
- 2 cups [300g] of green beans, trimmed
- 1 tbsp [15ml] of lemon juice
- 1 tsp of fresh parsley, chopped (for garnish)

Directions:

1. Preheat the oven to 400°F [200°C].
2. Place the fish fillets on a parchment-lined baking sheet. Drizzle with olive oil and sprinkle with oregano, thyme, and salt.
3. Bake the fish fillets in the preheated oven for 12-15 minutes or until they are opaque and easily flake with a fork.
4. While the fish bakes, steam the green beans. In a saucepan, bring about 1 inch of water to a simmer. Place the green beans in a steamer basket and cover. Steam for 6-7 minutes or until tender but still vibrant green.
5. Once the fish and green beans are cooked, drizzle the fish with lemon juice and garnish with fresh parsley.
6. Serve the oven-baked fish fillets alongside the steamed green beans.

Vegetables with Wild Rice and Fennel

Time: 45 minutes	Serving Size: 2 servings
Prep Time: 15 minutes	Cook Time: 30 minutes

Each Serving Has:

Calories: 312, Carbohydrates: 45g, Saturated Fat: 1g, Protein: 7g, Fat: 12g, Sodium: 86mg, Potassium: 684mg, Fiber: 7g, Sugar: 6g, Vitamin C: 23mg, Calcium: 76mg, Iron: 3mg

Ingredients:

- 1/2 cup [95g] rinsed wild rice
- 1 1/2 cups [360ml] water
- 1 tbsp olive oil
- 1 cup [110g] thinly sliced fennel bulb
- 1/2 cup [65g] peeled and diced carrot
- 1/2 cup [75g] chopped zucchini
- 1/2 cup [80g] diced cooked sweet potato
- 1/4 cup [60ml] low-sodium vegetable broth
- 1 tbsp chopped fresh dill
- 1/8 tsp sea salt (optional)

Directions:

1. Boil water in a small saucepan. Stir in wild rice, cover, and simmer 30–35 minutes until tender and absorbed. Let sit, covered.
2. Heat the olive oil in a large nonstick skillet over medium heat.
3. Add the sliced fennel bulb, diced carrot, and chopped zucchini to the skillet. Sauté for 5 minutes, stirring occasionally, until the vegetables begin to soften.
4. Add the diced sweet potato and vegetable broth to the skillet. Reduce the heat to low, cover, and let the vegetables braise gently for 10 minutes, or until all are tender.
5. Remove the lid and stir in the chopped dill and sea salt (if using). Cook for another minute.
6. Fluff the cooked wild rice with a fork and divide evenly between two plates. Top each with the braised vegetable mixture and serve.

Poached Chicken with Asparagus and Parsley

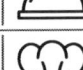 Time: 30 minutes	Serving Size: 2 plates
Prep Time: 10 minutes	Cook Time: 20 minutes

Each Serving Has:

Calories: 300, Carbohydrates: 8g, Saturated Fat: 1g, Protein: 38g, Fat: 9g, Sodium: 180mg, Potassium: 800mg, Fiber: 3g, Sugar: 3g, Vitamin C: 15mg, Calcium: 45mg, Iron: 2mg.

Ingredients:

- 2 boneless, skinless chicken breasts (about 8 oz [227g] each)
- 1 tbsp [15ml] of olive oil
- 1/2 cup [120ml] of low-sodium chicken broth
- 1 tsp of dried thyme
- 1/4 tsp of salt
- 1 bunch of asparagus, trimmed and cut into 2-inch pieces
- 1 tbsp of fresh parsley, chopped (for garnish)

Directions:

1. Heat olive oil in a skillet over medium heat. Season the chicken breasts with salt and thyme, then cook for 4-5 minutes per side until lightly browned.
2. Once the chicken is browned, add the chicken broth to the skillet. Cover and let simmer for 10-12 minutes, or until the chicken is fully cooked through.
3. While the chicken cooks, bring a small pot of water to a boil. Blanch the asparagus for 2-3 minutes until tender-crisp, then drain and set aside.
4. Once the chicken is done, remove it from the skillet and slice it into thin strips.
5. In the same skillet, add the cooked asparagus and a bit more chicken broth or water if needed. Stir for 1-2 minutes to combine the flavors.
6. Plate the sliced chicken alongside the asparagus and sprinkle with fresh parsley.

Lentil and Cabbage Stew with Sweet Potatoes

Time: 50 minutes	Serving Size: 2 servings
Prep Time: 15 minutes	Cook Time: 35 minutes

Each Serving Has:

Calories: 328, Carbohydrates: 53g, Saturated Fat: 1g, Protein: 13g, Fat: 9g, Sodium: 92mg, Potassium: 942mg, Fiber: 13g, Sugar: 9g, Vitamin C: 41mg, Calcium: 86mg, Iron: 4mg

Ingredients:

- 1/2 cup [100g] rinsed green lentils
- 3 cups [720ml] water
- 1 tbsp olive oil
- 1 cup [90g] shredded green cabbage
- 1/2 cup [75g] peeled and diced
- carrot
- 1 cup [160g] peeled and cubed sweet potato
- 1/2 cup [80g] diced zucchini
- 1 tbsp chopped fresh parsley
- 1/8 tsp sea salt (optional)

Directions:

1. In a medium saucepan, bring the water to a boil over high heat. Stir in the green lentils, reduce the heat to low, cover, and simmer for 25 minutes, or until just tender.
2. While the lentils cook, heat the olive oil in a large pot over medium heat.
3. Add the shredded green cabbage, diced carrot, cubed sweet potato, and diced zucchini to the pot. Stir well and cook for 5 minutes, allowing the vegetables to begin softening.
4. Once the lentils are cooked, transfer them along with any remaining cooking liquid into the pot with the vegetables.
5. Stir the mixture, cover, and let it simmer on low heat for 10–12 minutes, until the sweet potatoes are tender and the stew has thickened.
6. Stir in the chopped parsley and sea salt (if using). Let sit for 2 minutes, then serve warm.

Wild Rice and Mushroom Casserole

 Time:
40 minutes

 Serving Size:
2 bowls

 Prep Time:
10 minutes

 Cook Time:
30 minutes

Each Serving Has:

Calories: 310, Carbohydrates: 52g, Saturated Fat: 2g, Protein: 9g, Fat: 7g, Sodium: 280mg, Potassium: 400mg, Fiber: 6g, Sugar: 3g, Vitamin C: 4mg, Calcium: 60mg, Iron: 3mg.

Ingredients:
- 1/2 cup [90g] of wild rice
- 1 cup [70g] of mushrooms, sliced
- 1 tbsp [15ml] of olive oil
- 1 small onion, finely chopped
- 1 garlic clove, minced (optional)
- 1/2 cup [120ml] of vegetable broth
- 1/4 cup [60ml] of low-fat milk
- 1 tbsp of fresh thyme, chopped
- 1 tbsp of fresh parsley, chopped
- 1/4 tsp of salt
- 1/4 cup of grated reduced-fat Parmesan cheese [20g] (optional)

Directions:

1. Cook the wild rice according to package instructions.
2. Preheat the oven to 375°F [190°C].
3. In a skillet, heat olive oil over medium heat. Add onion and cook for about 4 minutes, until softened.
4. Add the mushrooms and garlic (if using) to the skillet. Cook for another 5-7 minutes, stirring occasionally, until the mushrooms soften.
5. Add the broth, milk, thyme, parsley, and salt to the skillet. Stir, bring to a simmer, and cook for 3-4 minutes.
6. Once the rice is cooked, add it to the skillet with the mushroom mixture and stir until well combined.
7. Transfer the mixture to a greased baking dish and sprinkle with grated Parmesan (if using).
8. Bake the casserole in the oven for 15-20 minutes until the top is golden.
9. Let cool slightly before serving.

Baked Sweet Bell Peppers with Millet and Herbs

 Time:
55 minutes

 Serving Size:
2 servings

 Prep Time:
20 minutes

 Cook Time:
35 minutes

Each Serving Has:

Calories: 298, Carbohydrates: 45g, Saturated Fat: 1g, Protein: 8g, Fat: 10g, Sodium: 57mg, Potassium: 678mg, Fiber: 7g, Sugar: 8g, Vitamin C: 142mg, Calcium: 52mg, Iron: 2mg

Ingredients:
- 1/2 cup [90g] rinsed millet
- 1 1/2 cups [360ml] water
- 1/2 tsp olive oil
- 2 medium yellow bell peppers, halved lengthwise and seeds removed
- 1/2 cup [75g] chopped zucchini
- 1/2 cup [80g] chopped peeled carrot
- 1/4 cup [60ml] unsweetened oat milk
- 1 tbsp chopped fresh parsley
- 1 tsp chopped fresh dill
- 1/8 tsp sea salt (optional)

Directions:

1. Preheat the oven to 375°F [190°C].
2. Boil water in a medium saucepan. Stir in millet, cover, and simmer on low for 20 minutes until tender and absorbed. Set aside.
3. Heat the olive oil in a skillet over medium-low heat.
4. Sauté the chopped zucchini and carrot for 5–6 minutes, stirring often, until softened but not browned.
5. In a bowl, combine the cooked millet, sautéed vegetables, oat milk, chopped parsley, dill, and sea salt (if using). Stir thoroughly to form a moist filling.
6. Place the halved yellow bell peppers, cut side up, in a baking dish.
7. Spoon the millet mixture evenly into each pepper half, gently pressing to fill.
8. Cover the baking dish with foil and bake for 25 minutes.
9. Remove the foil and bake for an additional 10 minutes, until the peppers are tender and the tops lightly golden.
10. Let cool slightly before serving warm.

Lentil and Cauliflower Casserole

 Time:
45 minutes

 Serving Size:
2 bowls

Prep Time:
15 minutes

Cook Time:
30 minutes

Each Serving Has:
Calories: 320, Carbohydrates: 40g, Saturated Fat: 2g, Protein: 15g, Fat: 12g, Sodium: 250mg, Potassium: 800mg, Fiber: 12g, Sugar: 8g, Vitamin C: 85mg, Calcium: 150mg, Iron: 3mg.

Ingredients:
- 1/2 cup of dried lentils [3.5 oz / 100g], rinsed
- 1 small cauliflower [about 1 lb / 450g], cut into florets
- 1 tbsp of olive oil [15ml]
- 1 small onion [about 4 oz / 115g], finely chopped
- 1/2 cup [120ml]
- of low-sodium vegetable broth
- 1/4 tsp of ground turmeric
- 1/4 tsp of ground cumin
- 1/4 tsp of paprika
- 1/8 tsp of salt
- 1 tbsp of fresh parsley, chopped (for garnish)

Directions:
1. Preheat the oven to 375°F [190°C].
2. In a saucepan, bring 2 cups (475ml) of water to a boil. Add the lentils and cook for 20–25 minutes, or until tender. Drain any excess water and set aside.
3. While the lentils cook, heat the olive oil in a skillet over medium heat. Add the onion and cook for 4-5 minutes.
4. Add the cauliflower to the skillet and stir with onions. Cook for about 5-7 minutes, until the cauliflower is just tender.
5. Stir in lentils, broth, turmeric, cumin, paprika, and salt. Mix well and cook for an another 5 minutes.
6. Transfer the lentil and cauliflower mixture to a baking dish, spread evenly, and bake in the oven for 20-25 minutes until the cauliflower is fully tender and the top is golden.
7. Remove from the oven, cool slightly, and garnish with parsley.

Pumpkin and Chickpea Stew

 Time:
40 minutes

Serving Size:
2 bowls

 Prep Time:
10 minutes

 Cook Time:
30 minutes

Each Serving Has:
Calories: 320, Carbohydrates: 45g, Saturated Fat: 1g, Protein: 10g, Fat: 12g, Sodium: 250mg, Potassium: 900mg, Fiber: 12g, Sugar: 9g, Vitamin C: 18mg, Calcium: 80mg, Iron: 3mg.

Ingredients:
- 1/2 lb [227g] of pumpkin, peeled and cubed
- 1 cup [170g] of cooked chickpeas (or 1 can, drained and rinsed)
- 1 tbsp of olive oil [15ml]
- 1 small onion [about 4 oz / 115g], chopped
- 1 garlic clove, minced (optional)
- 1 tsp of ground cumin
- 1/2 tsp of ground
- coriander
- 1/4 tsp of ground turmeric
- 1/4 tsp of ground cinnamon
- 2 cups [475ml] of low-sodium vegetable broth
- 1/2 cup [120ml] of coconut milk
- 1 tbsp offresh lemon juice
- 2 tbsp of fresh parsley, chopped (for garnish)
- 1/8 tsp of salt

Directions:
1. Heat olive oil in a pot over medium heat. Add the onion and cook for 4-5 minutes until softened.
2. Add the garlic (if using) and cook for 1 minute, stirring constantly.
3. Add the pumpkin to the pot and cook for 5-7 minutes, stirring occasionally, until slightly tender.
4. Sprinkle in cumin, coriander, turmeric, cinnamon and salt. Stir well.
5. Pour in the broth, bring to a boil, then reduce heat and simmer for 15-20 minutes, until the pumpkin is tender.
6. Stir in the cooked chickpeas and coconut milk, and cook for an another 5 minutes.
7. Add lemon juice to the stew and garnish with parsley.

Shrimp with Rice Noodles and Bok Choy

 Time:
35 minutes

 Serving Size:
2 servings

 Prep Time:
15 minutes

Cook Time:
20 minutes

Each Serving Has:
Calories: 312, Carbohydrates: 38g, Saturated Fat: 0.5g, Protein: 24g, Fat: 8g, Sodium: 162mg, Potassium: 680mg, Fiber: 4g, Sugar: 3g, Vitamin C: 52mg, Calcium: 108mg, Iron: 3mg

Ingredients:
- 4 oz [115g] peeled and deveined raw medium shrimp
- 4 oz [115g] dried rice noodles
- 2 cups [150g] chopped bok choy
- 1 tbsp chopped fresh parsley
- 1/2 tsp chopped fresh dill
- 1 tsp olive oil
- 1/8 tsp sea salt (optional)

Directions:
1. Soak the rice noodles in warm water for 10 minutes, then drain and set aside.
2. Prepare a steamer setup and bring the water to a gentle boil over medium heat.
3. Place the chopped bok choy in the steamer basket and steam for 7–8 minutes until tender but still vibrant.
4. Remove the bok choy and set aside. Place the shrimp in the steamer basket and steam for 5–6 minutes, or until they are pink and cooked through.
5. In a large sauté pan over low heat, warm the olive oil.
6. Add the softened rice noodles to the pan and gently toss with the steamed shrimp, bok choy, chopped parsley, dill, and sea salt (if using). Stir to combine evenly and heat through for 1–2 minutes.
7. Divide the mixture between two plates and serve warm.

Rice and Zucchini Casserole with Soft Tofu

 Time:
50 minutes

 Serving Size:
2 servings

 Prep Time:
15 minutes

 Cook Time:
35 minutes

Each Serving Has:
Calories: 312, Carbohydrates: 42g, Saturated Fat: 0.8g, Protein: 13g, Fat: 10g, Sodium: 150mg, Potassium: 580mg, Fiber: 4g, Sugar: 4g, Vitamin C: 22mg, Calcium: 240mg, Iron: 2.1mg

Ingredients:
- 1 cup [195g] cooked brown rice
- 1 1/2 cups [180g] grated zucchini
- 1/2 cup [120g] mashed soft tofu
- 1/2 cup [120ml] unsweetened
- almond milk
- 1 tbsp chopped fresh parsley
- 1 tbsp chopped fresh dill
- 1 tbsp nutritional yeast
- 1/2 tsp olive oil

Directions:
1. Preheat the oven to 350°F [175°C]. Lightly grease a small baking dish with olive oil.
2. In a large bowl, combine cooked brown rice, grated zucchini, mashed tofu, almond milk, chopped parsley, dill, and nutritional yeast.
3. Stir the mixture thoroughly until well combined and evenly moistened.
4. Transfer the mixture into the greased baking dish and spread it evenly.
5. Cover the dish with foil and bake for 25 minutes.
6. Remove the foil and bake for an additional 10 minutes until the top is slightly firm and the edges are lightly golden.
7. Let the casserole rest for 5 minutes before serving warm.

Roasted Carrot and Fennel Bake

Time: 45 minutes	**Serving Size:** 2 servings
Prep Time: 15 minutes	**Cook Time:** 30 minutes

Each Serving Has:
Calories: 200, Carbohydrates: 38g, Saturated Fat: 2g, Protein: 4g, Fat: 7g, Sodium: 180mg, Potassium: 650mg, Fiber: 7g, Sugar: 10g, Vitamin C: 15mg, Calcium: 80mg, Iron: 2mg.

Ingredients:
- 2 large carrots, peeled and sliced into rounds (about 1 cup [130g])
- 1 medium fennel bulb, trimmed and sliced thinly (about 1 cup [100g])
- 1 tbsp [15ml] of olive oil
- 1 tsp of dried thyme
- 1/2 tsp of garlic powder
- 1/6 tsp of salt
- 1/2 cup [50g] of whole wheat breadcrumbs
- 1/4 cup [30g] of grated reduced-fat Parmesan cheese
- 1 tbsp of fresh parsley, chopped (for garnish)

Directions:
1. Preheat the oven to 375°F (190°C).
2. In a bowl, toss the carrots and fennel with olive oil, thyme, garlic powder, and salt. Toss the vegetables to coat evenly with the seasoning and oil.
3. Spread the seasoned carrots and fennel on a lined baking sheet.
4. Roast the vegetables in the preheated oven for 20 minutes, stirring halfway through to ensure even cooking.
5. After 20 minutes, remove the baking sheet from the oven and sprinkle the vegetables with breadcrumbs and Parmesan.
6. Roast for another 10 minutes, or until the vegetables are tender and golden brown.
7. Remove from the oven and allow to cool slightly. Garnish with parsley before serving.

Steamed Halibut with Parsley and Wild Rice

Time: 30 minutes	**Serving Size:** 2 plates
Prep Time: 10 minutes	**Cook Time:** 20 minutes

Each Serving Has:
Calories: 350, Carbohydrates: 34g, Saturated Fat: 1g, Protein: 32g, Fat: 9g, Sodium: 120mg, Potassium: 950mg, Fiber: 4g, Sugar: 2g, Vitamin C: 20mg, Calcium: 50mg, Iron: 3mg.

Ingredients:
- 2 halibut fillets (about 6 oz [170g] each)
- 1/2 cup [90g] of wild rice
- 1 tbsp [15ml] of olive oil
- 1 lemon, thinly sliced
- 1/4 tsp of garlic powder
- 1/8 tsp of ground black pepper (optional)
- 1/8 tsp of salt
- 1 1/2 [360ml] cups of water
- 1/4 cup [5g] of fresh parsley, chopped (for garnish)

Directions:
1. Rinse the wild rice, then combine with water in a saucepan. Bring to a boil, reduce heat, cover, and simmer for 15-20 minutes until tender. Fluff with a fork and set aside.
2. While the rice cooks, season the halibut fillets with garlic powder, black pepper (if using), and salt. Place the fillets on a heatproof plate.
3. Fill a large pot with a couple of inches of water and bring to a simmer. Place a steaming rack or basket in the pot, ensuring the water doesn't touch the fillets. Arrange the halibut in the basket, top with lemon slices, cover, and steam for 8-10 minutes, until the fish flakes easily with a fork.
4. Once the halibut is done, drizzle the fillets with olive oil.
5. Serve the steamed halibut over a bed of wild rice, garnished with parsley.

Baked Chicken with Herb Sauce

Time: 40 minutes	Serving Size: 2 plates
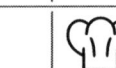 Prep Time: 10 minutes	Cook Time: 30 minutes

Each Serving Has:
Calories: 350, Carbohydrates: 10g, Saturated Fat: 1g, Protein: 40g, Fat: 15g, Sodium: 220mg, Potassium: 500mg, Fiber: 2g, Sugar: 4g, Vitamin C: 10mg, Calcium: 40mg, Iron: 2mg.

Ingredients:
- 2 boneless, skinless chicken breasts (6 oz [170g] each)
- 2 tbsp [30ml] of olive oil
- 1 tbsp [5g] of fresh rosemary, chopped
- 1 tbsp [5g] of fresh thyme, chopped
- 1 tsp [3g] of garlic powder
- 1/2 cup [120ml] of low-sodium vegetable broth
- 1/2 cup [120ml] of unsweetened almond milk
- 1 tbsp [15ml] of Dijon mustard
- 1 tbsp [3g] of fresh parsley, chopped
- 1 tbsp [15ml] of olive oil for drizzling

Directions:
1. Preheat the oven to 375°F [190°C].
2. Place chicken breasts on a baking sheet, drizzle with olive oil, and season with garlic powder, rosemary, and thyme. Massage the seasoning into the chicken.
3. Bake the chicken in the oven for 25-30 minutes, until the chicken is fully cooked.
4. While the chicken bakes, prepare the herb sauce. In a saucepan, combine the broth, almond milk, Dijon mustard, and parsley. Simmer over medium heat for 5-7 minutes, stirring occasionally, until the sauce thickens slightly.
5. Once the chicken is done, remove it from the oven and let it rest for 5 minutes.
6. Drizzle the warm herb sauce over the chicken breasts and serve.

Turkey Breast with Millet and Pumpkin Puree

Time: 55 minutes	Serving Size: 2 servings
Prep Time: 15 minutes	Cook Time: 40 minutes

Each Serving Has:
Calories: 346, Carbohydrates: 29g, Saturated Fat: 1g, Protein: 33g, Fat: 11g, Sodium: 122mg, Potassium: 758mg, Fiber: 4g, Sugar: 4g, Vitamin C: 9mg, Calcium: 34mg, Iron: 2.6mg

Ingredients:
- 2 cups [480ml] water
- 1/2 cup [85g] rinsed millet
- 2 tsp olive oil
- 2 pieces [150g each] skinless turkey breast fillet
- 1/2 tsp dried thyme
- 1/4 tsp sea salt (optional)
- 1 1/2 cups [340g] mashed cooked pumpkin
- 1/2 cup [120ml] unsweetened almond milk

Directions:
1. Preheat the oven to 375°F [190°C]. Grease a baking dish with 1 teaspoon of olive oil.
2. Rub turkey breast fillets with dried thyme, sea salt (if using), and 1 teaspoon of olive oil. Place the turkey in the baking dish.
3. Bake the turkey uncovered for 35–40 minutes, or until tender and cooked.
4. Boil water in a small saucepan. Add rinsed millet, cover, and simmer on low for 18–20 minutes until fluffy and absorbed. Remove from heat and let sit, covered.
5. In a small saucepan over low heat, combine mashed cooked pumpkin and almond milk. Stir the mixture frequently for 5 minutes, until it is warmed through and smooth.
6. Divide the cooked millet between two plates, spoon the pumpkin puree alongside, and top with oven-baked turkey breast. Serve warm.

Sweet Potato and Fennel Gratin

 Time: 55 minutes

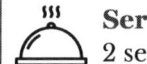 **Serving Size:** 2 servings

Prep Time: 15 minutes

Cook Time: 40 minutes

Each Serving Has:
Calories: 248, Carbohydrates: 39g, Saturated Fat: 1g, Protein: 3g, Fat: 10g, Sodium: 112mg, Potassium: 765mg, Fiber: 6g, Sugar: 8g, Vitamin C: 24mg, Calcium: 82mg, Iron: 1.2mg

Ingredients:
- 1 tbsp olive oil
- 1 1/2 cups [225g] peeled and thinly sliced sweet potato
- 1 cup [90g] thinly sliced fennel bulb
- 1/2 cup [120ml] unsweetened oat
- milk
- 1/4 cup [60ml] water
- 1 tsp chopped fresh parsley
- 1/8 tsp sea salt (optional)

Directions:
1. Preheat the oven to 375°F [190°C]. Lightly grease a small baking dish with olive oil.
2. Layer half of the sliced sweet potato in the bottom of the prepared baking dish.
3. Arrange all of the sliced fennel bulb evenly over the sweet potato layer.
4. Layer the remaining sweet potato slices on top of the fennel.
5. In a small bowl, whisk together oat milk, water, chopped parsley, and sea salt (if using) until well combined.
6. Pour the oat milk mixture evenly over the layered vegetables in the baking dish.
7. Cover the dish with foil and bake for 30 minutes.
8. Remove the foil and continue baking for an additional 10 minutes, until the top is lightly golden and the vegetables are tender.
9. Let rest for 5 minutes before serving.

Lentil and Wild Rice Casserole

 Time: 1 hour 15 minutes

 Serving Size: 2 bowls

Prep Time: 15 minutes

Cook Time: 1 hour

Each Serving Has:
Calories: 350, Carbohydrates: 60g, Saturated Fat: 1g, Protein: 14g, Fat: 6g, Sodium: 200mg, Potassium: 800mg, Fiber: 12g, Sugar: 5g, Vitamin C: 20mg, Calcium: 50mg, Iron: 3mg.

Ingredients:
- 1/2 cup [100g] of dry lentils
- 1/2 cup [85g] of wild rice
- 2 tbsp [30ml] of olive oil
- 1 small onion, diced
- 1 medium carrot, peeled and diced
- 1 tsp of ground cumin
- 1/2 tsp of turmeric
- 1/2 tsp of dried thyme
- 1 cup [240ml] of low-sodium vegetable broth
- 1/2 cup [120ml] of water
- 1/8 tsp of salt
- 1/4 cup of fresh parsley, chopped (for garnish)

Directions:
1. Preheat the oven to 375°F [190°C].
2. Rinse the lentils and wild rice under cold water and drain well.
3. Heat 1 tbsp olive oil in a pot over medium heat. Add onion and carrot, sauté for 4-5.
4. Stir in the cumin, turmeric, and thyme, cooking for another minute.
5. Add the lentils, rice, broth, and water to the pot. Bring to a boil, then reduce heat to low. Cover and simmer for 30 minutes, or until tender.
6. Heat the remaining olive oil in a skillet over medium heat. Add the rice and lentils, stir to combine, and season with salt.
7. Transfer to a greased baking dish, cover with foil, and bake for 25 minutes.
8. Fluff with a fork and garnish with parsley before serving.

Cauliflower and Spinach Bake

 Time: 45 minutes

 Serving Size: 2 bowls

 Prep Time: 15 minutes

Cook Time: 30 minutes

Each Serving Has:
Calories: 220, Carbohydrates: 20g, Saturated Fat: 2g, Protein: 10g, Fat: 12g, Sodium: 250mg, Potassium: 680mg, Fiber: 8g, Sugar: 5g, Vitamin C: 45mg, Calcium: 150mg, Iron: 2mg.

Ingredients:
- 1/2 medium cauliflower, cut into florets
- 2 cups [60g] of fresh spinach
- 1/2 cup [120g] of low-fat ricotta cheese
- 1/4 cup [30g] of grated reduced-fat Parmesan cheese
- 1 tbsp [15ml] of olive oil
- 1/4 tsp of ground nutmeg
- 1/4 tsp of garlic powder
- 1/2 tsp of dried oregano
- 1 tbsp of chopped fresh basil
- 1/8 tsp of salt

Directions:
1. Preheat the oven to 375°F [190°C].
2. Steam the cauliflower in a steamer basket over boiling water for 7-10 minutes, or boil in a pot for 7-10 minutes. Drain well and set aside.
3. Heat the olive oil in a skillet over medium heat. Add the spinach and sauté until wilted, about 2-3 minutes. Set aside.
4. In a mixing bowl, combine the ricotta, Parmesan, nutmeg, garlic powder, oregano, basil, and salt. Mix until well combined.
5. Add the cooked cauliflower and spinach to the cheese mixture. Stir gently until the vegetables are evenly coated.
6. Transfer the mixture to a lightly greased baking dish.
7. Bake the casserole in the oven for 20-25 minutes, until the top is lightly golden.
8. Remove from the oven and let cool slightly before serving.

White Fish with Barley and Carrot Puree

 Time: 55 minutes

 Serving Size: 2 servings

 Prep Time: 15 minutes

 Cook Time: 40 minutes

Each Serving Has:
Calories: 328, Carbohydrates: 38g, Saturated Fat: 1g, Protein: 28g, Fat: 9g, Sodium: 112mg, Potassium: 987mg, Fiber: 6g, Sugar: 6g, Vitamin C: 14mg, Calcium: 55mg, Iron: 2.3mg

Ingredients:
- 1/2 cup [100g] rinsed pearl barley
- 1 1/2 cups [360ml] water
- 1 1/2 cups [180g] peeled and sliced carrots
- 1/2 cup [120ml] unsweetened oat milk
- 1/2 tsp olive oil
- 2 fillets [200g] skinless white fish (such as cod or tilapia)
- 2 cups [480ml] low-sodium vegetable broth
- 1 tbsp chopped fresh dill
- 1/8 tsp sea salt (optional)

Directions:
1. Combine pearl barley and water in a medium saucepan. Bring to a boil over medium heat, then reduce heat to low, cover, and simmer 30 minutes until tender and water is absorbed.
2. Place sliced carrots in a separate saucepan and cover with water. Bring to a gentle boil and cook for 15–20 minutes until very soft.
3. Drain the cooked carrots and transfer them to a blender. Add oat milk, olive oil, and sea salt (if using). Blend until smooth and creamy. Set aside, keeping warm.
4. In a wide, shallow pan, bring the vegetable broth to a gentle simmer over low heat. Carefully place the white fish fillets into the broth and poach for 8–10 minutes until flaky.
5. Divide the cooked barley between two plates. Spoon the carrot puree alongside the barley, and place a poached fish fillet on top.
6. Sprinkle with chopped dill and serve.

Roasted Pumpkin and Mushroom Bowl

Time: 35 minutes	Serving Size: 2 bowls
Prep Time: 10 minutes	Cook Time: 25 minutes

Each Serving Has:

Calories: 220, Carbohydrates: 40g, Saturated Fat: 1g, Protein: 6g, Fat: 4g, Sodium: 150mg, Potassium: 650mg, Fiber: 8g, Sugar: 8g, Vitamin C: 20mg, Calcium: 60mg, Iron: 3mg.

Ingredients:

- 1 small pumpkin [1 lb / 453.6g], peeled and diced
- 8 oz [227g] of button mushrooms, cleaned and sliced
- 1 tbsp [15ml] of olive oil
- 1/4 tsp of ground cumin
- 1/4 tsp of ground turmeric
- 1/2 tsp of garlic powder
- 1/8 tsp of salt
- 1 cup [185g] of cooked quinoa
- 2 tbsp of fresh parsley, chopped (for garnish)
- 1 tbsp of pumpkin seeds (for garnish)

Directions:

1. Preheat the oven to 400°F [200°C].
2. In a mixing bowl, toss the pumpkin and mushrooms with olive oil, cumin, turmeric, garlic powder, and salt. Ensure all the vegetables are well-coated.
3. Spread the pumpkin and mushroom mixture on a baking sheet. Roast in the oven for 20-25 minutes, flipping halfway through, until the pumpkin is tender and the mushrooms are golden.
4. While the vegetables are roasting, cook the quinoa according to the package instructions. Once cooked, fluff with a fork and set aside.
5. Once the vegetables are done, remove them from the oven and set aside to cool slightly.
6. Serve the cooked quinoa topped with the roasted pumpkin and mushrooms.
7. Sprinkle parsley and pumpkin seeds on top.

Herb-Roasted Vegetables with Brown Rice

Time: 45 minutes	Serving Size: 2 bowls
Prep Time: 15 minutes	Cook Time: 30 minutes

Each Serving Has:

Calories: 330, Carbohydrates: 58g, Saturated Fat: 1g, Protein: 8g, Fat: 6g, Sodium: 150mg, Potassium: 890mg, Fiber: 10g, Sugar: 9g, Vitamin C: 45mg, Calcium: 60mg, Iron: 3mg.

Ingredients:

- 1 cup [185g] of cooked brown rice
- 1 medium zucchini [200g], sliced into half-moons
- 1 medium carrot [70g], peeled and cut into rounds
- 1 small sweet potato [180g], peeled and cubed
- 1 tbsp [15ml] of olive oil
- 1/2 tsp of dried rosemary
- 1/2 tsp of dried thyme
- 1/4 tsp of garlic powder
- 1/8 tsp of salt
- 2 tbsp of fresh parsley, chopped (for garnish)

Directions:

1. Preheat the oven to 400°F [200°C].
2. In a bowl, combine the zucchini, carrot, and sweet potato. Drizzle with olive oil and toss to coat the vegetables.
3. Sprinkle the vegetables with rosemary, thyme, garlic powder, and salt. Toss again to evenly distribute the seasonings.
4. Spread the seasoned vegetables in a single layer on a baking sheet. Roast for 25-30 minutes, flipping halfway, until tender and slightly golden brown.
5. While the vegetables are roasting, cook the brown rice according to the package instructions. Once cooked, fluff the rice with a fork and set aside.
6. Remove the roasted vegetables from the oven and let them cool slightly.
7. Serve the cooked brown rice topped with the roasted vegetables and sprinkle with parsley.

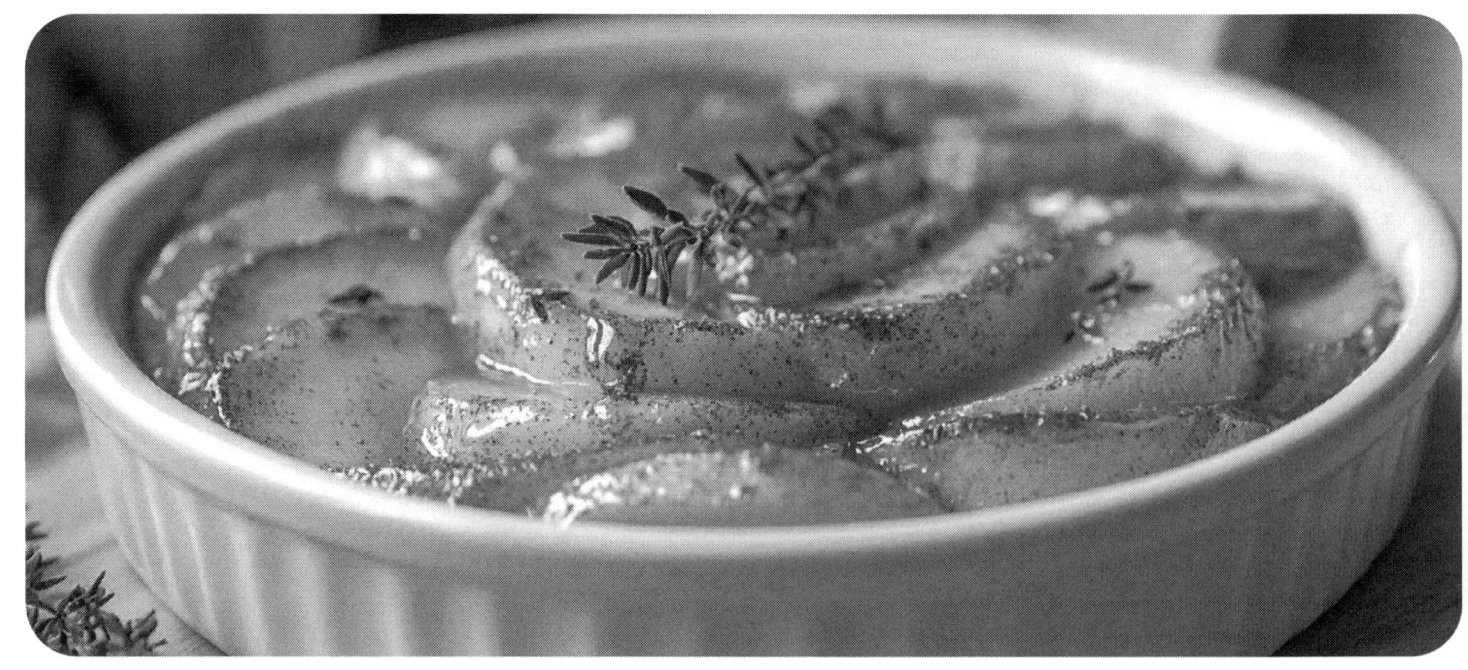

Chapter 7: Desserts

Baked Quince with Rice and Cinnamon

Time: 1 hour 5 minutes	**Serving Size:** 2 servings
Prep Time: 20 minutes	**Cook Time:** 45 minutes

Each Serving Has:
Calories: 285, Carbohydrates: 58g, Saturated Fat: 0.5g, Protein: 4g, Fat: 4g, Sodium: 8mg, Potassium: 412mg, Fiber: 5g, Sugar: 21g, Vitamin C: 18mg, Calcium: 35mg, Iron: 1.2mg

Ingredients:
- 2 medium quinces, peeled, cored, and halved
- 1 tbsp maple syrup
- 1/2 tsp ground cinnamon
- 1/4 tsp ground ginger
- 1 tsp olive oil
- 1/2 cup [90g] rinsed brown rice
- 1 1/2 cups [360ml] water
- 1/4 cup [60ml] unsweetened almond milk
- 1 tbsp chopped soft dates
- 1/2 tsp vanilla extract

Directions:
1. Preheat the oven to 350°F [175°C].
2. In a small saucepan, combine brown rice and water. Bring to a boil, then reduce the heat to low, cover, and simmer for 35–40 minutes, or until the rice is tender and the water is absorbed.
3. While the rice cooks, place halved quinces in a small baking dish. Drizzle with maple syrup and olive oil, then sprinkle with ground cinnamon and ground ginger.
4. Cover the baking dish tightly with foil and bake in the preheated oven for 40–45 minutes, or until the quinces are soft and lightly caramelized.
5. In a small bowl, combine the cooked brown rice, almond milk, chopped dates, and vanilla extract. Stir well to blend into a creamy mixture.
6. To serve, place one baked quince half on each plate and spoon half of the rice mixture into the center cavity. Serve warm.

Low-Sugar Zucchini Bread

 Time:
1 hour 15 minutes

 Serving Size:
2 servings

 Prep Time:
15 minutes

Cook Time:
1 hour

Each Serving Has:

Calories: 180, Carbohydrates: 32g, Saturated Fat: 1g, Protein: 4g, Fat: 7g, Sodium: 150mg, Potassium: 350mg, Fiber: 4g, Sugar: 8g, Vitamin C: 4mg, Calcium: 40mg, Iron: 1.5mg.

Ingredients:

- 1 cup [130g] of shredded zucchini
- 1/2 cup [56g] of almond flour
- 1/2 cup [60g] of whole wheat flour
- 1/4 cup [60ml] of unsweetened applesauce
- 1/4 cup [60ml] of pure maple syrup
- 2 large eggs
- 1 tsp of vanilla extract
- 1/2 tsp of ground cinnamon
- 1/4 tsp of ground nutmeg
- 1/2 tsp of baking soda
- 1/8 tsp of salt
- 1/4 cup [30g] of chopped walnuts (optional)

Directions:

1. Preheat the oven to 350°F [175°C].
2. Grease a loaf pan with a small amount of olive oil or line with parchment paper.
3. In a bowl, combine almond flour, whole wheat flour, baking soda, cinnamon, nutmeg, and salt. Stir to mix evenly.
4. In another bowl, whisk together the eggs, maple syrup, applesauce, and vanilla extract until smooth.
5. Add the zucchini to the wet ingredients and mix well to combine.
6. Gradually add dry ingredients to wet, stirring until combined. Fold in chopped walnuts, if using.
7. Pour the batter into the loaf pan, smoothing the top evenly.
8. Bake for 1 hour or until a toothpick inserted into the center comes out clean.
9. Cool the zucchini bread in the pan for 10 minutes, then transfer to a wire rack to cool completely.

Rice Pudding with Almond Milk

 Time:
40 minutes

 Serving Size:
2 bowls

 Prep Time:
5 minutes

 Cook Time:
35 minutes

Each Serving Has:

Calories: 220, Carbohydrates: 40g, Saturated Fat: 1g, Protein: 4g, Fat: 4g, Sodium: 100mg, Potassium: 160mg, Fiber: 2g, Sugar: 10g, Vitamin C: 0mg, Calcium: 250mg, Iron: 1mg.

Ingredients:

- 1/2 cup [95g] of white rice
- 2 cups [480ml] of unsweetened almond milk
- 1 tbsp [15ml] of maple syrup
- 1/2 tsp of vanilla extract
- 1/4 tsp of ground cinnamon
- 1 tbsp [12g] of chia seeds
- 1/4 cup [20g] of unsweetened shredded coconut
- 1/4 cup [30g] of sliced almonds (for garnish)

Directions:

1. Rinse the white rice under cold water to remove excess starch.
2. In a saucepan, combine the rice and almond milk. Bring to a simmer over medium heat, stirring occasionally.
3. Reduce the heat to low, cover, and cook for 25-30 minutes, or until the rice is tender and the liquid is absorbed, stirring occasionally.
4. Once the rice is cooked, stir in the maple syrup, vanilla extract, cinnamon, and chia seeds. Continue cooking on low for an additional 5 minutes, allowing the chia seeds to thicken the mixture.
5. Remove the saucepan from the heat. Stir in the shredded coconut.
6. Let the pudding cool for a few minutes before serving.
7. Eop each serving with sliced almonds for extra crunch.

Pumpkin Spice Custard with Flaxseed

 Time:
40 minutes

 Serving Size:
2 small bowls

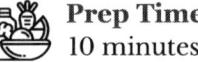 **Prep Time:**
10 minutes

 Cook Time:
30 minutes

Each Serving Has:
Calories: 180, Carbohydrates: 28g, Saturated Fat: 1g, Protein: 6g, Fat: 7g, Sodium: 50mg, Potassium: 300mg, Fiber: 6g, Sugar: 9g, Vitamin C: 5mg, Calcium: 80mg, Iron: 1.5mg.

Ingredients:
- 1/2 cup [120g] of canned pumpkin puree
- 1 cup [240ml] of unsweetened almond milk
- 1 tbsp [10g] of ground flaxseeds
- 1 tbsp [15ml] of maple syrup
- 1/2 tsp of ground cinnamon
- 1/4 tsp of ground ginger
- 1/4 tsp of ground nutmeg
- 1/2 tsp of vanilla extract
- 2 large eggs
- 1 tbsp [8g] of cornstarch
- 1/8 tsp of sea salt

Directions:
1. Preheat the oven to 350°F [175°C].
2. In a saucepan, combine almond milk, pumpkin puree, maple syrup, flaxseeds, cinnamon, ginger, nutmeg, vanilla extract, and salt. Stir over medium heat for about 5 minutes until warmed.
3. In a bowl, whisk the eggs and cornstarch until smooth. Gradually pour a small amount of the warm pumpkin mixture into the eggs, whisking constantly. Slowly add the egg mixture back into the saucepan, stirring continuously.
4. Continue cooking the mixture over medium-low heat, stirring frequently, until it thickens to a creamy consistency, about 10-12 minutes. Avoid boiling.
5. Once thickened, remove the saucepan from the heat. Pour the custard into two ramekins.
6. Cool the custard at room temperature for about 10 minutes, then refrigerate for at least 20 minutes.
7. Before serving, sprinkle a pinch of cinnamon on top.

Steamed Millet Pudding with Pear Compote

 Time:
50 minutes

 Serving Size:
2 servings

 Prep Time:
15 minutes

 Cook Time:
35 minutes

Each Serving Has:
Calories: 274, Carbohydrates: 49g, Saturated Fat: 0.6g, Protein: 6g, Fat: 6g, Sodium: 8mg, Potassium: 319mg, Fiber: 5g, Sugar: 15g, Vitamin C: 10mg, Calcium: 27mg, Iron: 1.4mg

Ingredients:
- 1/2 cup [90g] rinsed millet
- 1 1/2 cups [360ml] unsweetened oat milk
- 1 tbsp chopped soft dates
- 1/2 tsp ground cinnamon
- 1/2 tsp vanilla extract
- 1 tsp olive oil
- 2 medium pears, peeled, cored, and diced
- 2 tbsp water
- 1 tbsp maple syrup

Directions:
1. Grease the bottom and sides of a ceramic bowl with olive oil. Set aside.
2. Combine millet and oat milk in a saucepan. Simmer over medium-low heat, stirring occasionally.
3. Stir in chopped dates, cinnamon, and vanilla. Reduce heat to low, cover, and cook for 20–25 minutes, stirring occasionally, until millet is tender and mixture thickens.
4. Transfer the mixture to the greased bowl. Level the surface and place the bowl in a steamer over simmering water.
5. Cover and steam for 10 minutes, until the pudding is set and becomes creamy.
6. In a saucepan, combine diced pears and water. Cover and simmer on low for 10 minutes, stirring occasionally, until pears are soft and starting to break down.
7. Stir in the maple syrup and cook, uncovered, for 2–3 more minutes, until the mixture resembles a loose compote.
8. Remove the millet pudding from the steamer and let it rest for 5 minutes.

Spoon the pear compote over and serve.

Carrot and Oat Muffins

 Time:
40 minutes

 Serving Size:
2 muffins

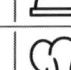 **Prep Time:**
15 minutes

Cook Time:
25 minutes

Each Serving Has:
Calories: 160, Carbohydrates: 28g, Saturated Fat: 1g, Protein: 3g, Fat: 5g, Sodium: 95mg, Potassium: 220mg, Fiber: 4g, Sugar: 9g, Vitamin C: 4mg, Calcium: 40mg, Iron: 1.2mg.

Ingredients:
- 1/2 cup [40g] of rolled oats
- 1/2 cup [60g] of whole wheat flour
- 1/2 tsp of baking soda
- 1/4 tsp of ground cinnamon
- 1/4 tsp of ground ginger
- 1/8 tsp of salt
- 1/4 cup of grated carrot
- 1/4 cup [60ml] of unsweetened applesauce
- 1 large egg
- 2 tbsp [30ml] of olive oil
- 2 tbsp [30ml] of maple syrup
- 1 tsp [5ml] of vanilla extract
- 2 tbsp [30ml] of unsweetened almond milk

Directions:
1. Preheat the oven to 350°F [175°C] and line a muffin tin with paper liners or lightly grease with olive oil.
2. In a bowl, combine the oats, whole wheat flour, baking soda, cinnamon, ginger, and salt. Stir to mix evenly.
3. In a separate bowl, whisk together the carrot, applesauce, egg, olive oil, maple syrup, vanilla extract, and almond milk until smooth.
4. Slowly add the wet ingredients to the dry, stirring gently to combine. The mixture should be thick, but moist.
5. Spoon the batter into the muffin tin, filling each muffin cup about 3/4 full.
6. Bake for 20-25 minutes or until a toothpick inserted into the center of a muffin comes out clean.
7. Cool the muffins in the tin for 5 minutes, then transfer to a wire rack to cool completely.

Baked Banana and Oat Squares

 Time:
40 minutes

 Serving Size:
2 servings

 Prep Time:
10 minutes

 Cook Time:
30 minutes

Each Serving Has:
Calories: 198, Carbohydrates: 33g, Saturated Fat: 0.4g, Protein: 4g, Fat: 5g, Sodium: 4mg, Potassium: 228mg, Fiber: 4g, Sugar: 9g, Vitamin C: 3mg, Calcium: 27mg, Iron: 1.1mg

Ingredients:
- 1/2 cup [45g] rolled oats
- 1/4 cup [60ml] unsweetened almond milk
- 1/4 medium banana, mashed [30g]
- 2 tbsp unsweetened
- applesauce
- 1 tbsp maple syrup
- 1/2 tsp ground cinnamon
- 1/4 tsp vanilla extract
- 1 tbsp chopped soft dates
- 1/2 tsp olive oil

Directions:
1. Preheat the oven to 350°F [175°C]. Lightly grease a small baking dish with olive oil.
2. In a medium bowl, combine mashed banana, almond milk, applesauce, maple syrup, ground cinnamon, vanilla extract, and chopped dates. Whisk until smooth and well incorporated.
3. Stir in rolled oats and mix until thoroughly combined. Let the mixture sit for 5 minutes to allow the oats to absorb moisture.
4. Pour the mixture into the prepared baking dish and smooth the top with a spatula.
5. Bake for 25–30 minutes, or until the edges are golden and the center is set.
6. Let cool for 10 minutes before slicing into squares. Serve warm.

Soft Baked Apple and Millet Muffins

Time: 40 minutes	Serving Size: 2 servings
Prep Time: 10 minutes	Cook Time: 30 minutes

Each Serving Has:
Calories: 213, Carbohydrates: 34g, Saturated Fat: 0.6g, Protein: 4g, Fat: 7g, Sodium: 42mg, Potassium: 186mg, Fiber: 3g, Sugar: 9g, Vitamin C: 3mg, Calcium: 28mg, Iron: 1.2mg

Ingredients:
- 1/4 cup [50g] cooked millet, cooled
- 1/2 cup [60g] grated peeled apple
- 1/4 cup [30g] oat flour
- 2 tbsp unsweetened applesauce
- 2 tbsp maple syrup
- 1 tbsp olive oil
- 1/4 tsp ground cinnamon
- 1/4 tsp baking soda
- 1/4 tsp vanilla extract
- 1 tbsp water

Directions:
1. Preheat the oven to 350°F [175°C]. Lightly grease two sections of a muffin tin with a small amount of olive oil or use paper liners.
2. In a medium bowl, combine grated apple, cooked millet, applesauce, maple syrup, olive oil, vanilla extract, and water. Stir until evenly mixed.
3. In a separate small bowl, whisk together oat flour, ground cinnamon, and baking soda.
4. Add the dry mixture to the wet ingredients and stir just until combined. Do not overmix.
5. Divide the batter evenly between the prepared muffin cups and smooth the tops.
6. Bake for 25–30 minutes, or until a toothpick inserted in the center comes out clean and the tops are firm to the touch.
7. Let the muffins cool in the pan for 5 minutes, then transfer to a wire rack to cool completely before serving.

Rice Pudding with Poached Peaches

Time: 45 minutes	Serving Size: 2 servings
Prep Time: 10 minutes	Cook Time: 35 minutes

Each Serving Has:
Calories: 214, Carbohydrates: 43g, Saturated Fat: 0.5g, Protein: 4g, Fat: 4g, Sodium: 36mg, Potassium: 246mg, Fiber: 2g, Sugar: 16g, Vitamin C: 7mg, Calcium: 89mg, Iron: 0.8mg

Ingredients:
- 1/4 cup [50g] uncooked short-grain white rice
- 1 1/2 cups [360ml] unsweetened oat milk
- 1 tbsp maple syrup
- 1/2 tsp vanilla
- extract
- 1/4 tsp ground cinnamon
- 2 medium ripe peaches, peeled, pitted, and sliced
- 1/2 cup [120ml] water

Directions:
1. In a medium saucepan, combine short-grain white rice and oat milk. Bring to a gentle simmer over medium heat.
2. Reduce the heat to low and cook, stirring occasionally, for 25–30 minutes, until the rice is tender and the mixture has thickened to a pudding-like consistency.
3. Stir in maple syrup, vanilla extract, and ground cinnamon. Continue cooking for 2 more minutes, then remove the pan from the heat and cover it to keep the food warm.
4. While the rice cooks, combine sliced peaches and water in a small saucepan.
5. Bring to a gentle simmer over medium-low heat, then cover and poach for 10–12 minutes, until the peaches are soft and translucent. Remove from heat.
6. Divide the rice pudding evenly between two bowls and top each with the warm poached peaches and a spoonful of their poaching liquid.
7. Serve warm or let cool slightly before serving.

Carrot and Millet Pudding with Cinnamon

 Time:
45 minutes

Serving Size:
2 servings

Prep Time:
10 minutes

Cook Time:
35 minutes

Each Serving Has:

Calories: 212, Carbohydrates: 36g, Saturated Fat: 0.6g, Protein: 5g, Fat: 5g, Sodium: 28mg, Potassium: 282mg, Fiber: 4g, Sugar: 10g, Vitamin C: 4mg, Calcium: 78mg, Iron: 1.3mg

Ingredients:

- 1/4 cup [48g] rinsed millet
- 1 cup [240ml] unsweetened oat milk
- 1/2 cup [60g] grated carrot
- 1 tbsp maple
- syrup
- 1/2 tsp ground cinnamon
- 1/4 tsp vanilla extract
- 1/4 tsp ground nutmeg
- 1/2 tsp olive oil

Directions:

1. Lightly grease a small saucepan with olive oil.
2. In the greased saucepan, combine rinsed millet and oat milk. Bring to a gentle simmer over medium heat.
3. Reduce the heat to low, cover, and cook for 20 minutes, stirring occasionally, until the millet begins to soften.
4. Stir in grated carrot, maple syrup, ground cinnamon, vanilla extract, and ground nutmeg.
5. Continue to simmer gently, uncovered, for 10–15 minutes, stirring frequently, until the mixture thickens to a soft pudding-like consistency and the carrots are fully tender.
6. Remove from heat and let sit for 5 minutes to allow the pudding to settle and slightly thicken.
7. Spoon the pudding into two small bowls and serve warm.

Applesauce and Oat Bars

 Time:
40 minutes

Serving Size:
2 bars

  Prep Time:
10 minutes

Cook Time:
30 minutes

Each Serving Has:

Calories: 180, Carbohydrates: 40g, Saturated Fat: 1g, Protein: 3g, Fat: 3g, Sodium: 15mg, Potassium: 160mg, Fiber: 4g, Sugar: 16g, Vitamin C: 2mg, Calcium: 25mg, Iron: 1mg.

Ingredients:

- 1 cup [240ml] of unsweetened applesauce
- 1/2 cup [45g] of rolled oats
- 1/4 cup [30g] of whole wheat flour
- 1/4 cup [60g] of unsweetened
- almond butter
- 1 tbsp [21g] of honey
- 1/2 tsp of ground cinnamon
- 1/4 tsp of vanilla extract
- Pinch of salt

Directions:

1. Preheat your oven to 350°F [175°C].
2. In a bowl, mix together the applesauce, almond butter, honey, and vanilla extract until smooth.
3. Add the oats, whole wheat flour, cinnamon, and a pinch of salt. Stir until everything is well combined into a thick batter.
4. Lightly grease a small baking dish (about 6x6 inches) with a bit of almond butter or non-stick spray.
5. Pour the batter into the prepared dish, spreading it evenly across the bottom.
6. Bake for 30 minutes, or until the bars are firm and lightly golden on top.
7. Allow the bars to cool in the dish for 10 minutes before cutting them into squares.

Baked Pumpkin and Oat Tartlets

 Time:
45 minutes

 Serving Size:
2 tartlets

 Prep Time:
15 minutes

 Cook Time:
30 minutes

Each Serving Has:
*Calories: 210, Carbohydrates: 28g, Saturated
Fat: 2g, Protein: 4g, Fat: 8g, Sodium: 70mg,
Potassium: 250mg, Fiber: 4g, Sugar: 9g,
Vitamin C: 12mg, Calcium: 30mg, Iron: 1mg.*

Ingredients:
- 1/2 cup [120g] of roasted pumpkin puree
- 1/4 cup [30g] of almond flour
- 2 tbsp [16g] of coconut flour
- 1 tbsp [21g] of honey
- 1 tsp of ground
- cinnamon
- 1/2 tsp of vanilla extract
- Pinch of salt
- 1 tbsp of coconut oil, melted
- 2 tbsp of almond milk
- 1/4 tsp of ground ginger

Directions:
1. Preheat the oven to 350°F [175°C].
2. In a bowl, combine the almond flour, coconut flour, cinnamon, ginger, and a pinch of salt.
3. Add the pumpkin puree, honey, almond milk, and vanilla extract to the dry ingredients. Stir until the mixture is smooth and well combined.
4. Divide the dough mixture evenly into two mini tartlet pans or muffin tins, pressing the dough down to form a crust at the bottom.
5. Place the tartlet pans in the oven and bake for about 25-30 minutes, or until the crust is golden and firm.
6. Remove from the oven and allow the tartlets to cool for 10 minutes before serving.

Sweet Potato Pie Bars

 Time:
50 minutes

Serving Size:
2 bars

 Prep Time:
15 minutes

Cook Time:
35 minutes

Each Serving Has:
*Calories: 180, Carbohydrates: 30g, Saturated
Fat: 2g, Protein: 3g, Fat: 6g, Sodium: 100mg,
Potassium: 400mg, Fiber: 5g, Sugar: 10g,
Vitamin C: 5mg, Calcium: 40mg, Iron: 1mg.*

Ingredients:
- 1/2 cup [120g] of mashed sweet potato
- 1/4 cup [30g] of almond flour
- 1/4 cup [24g] of rolled oats
- 2 tbsp [28g] of coconut oil, melted
- 1 tbsp [21g] of maple syrup
- 1/2 tsp of ground
- cinnamon
- 1/4 tsp of ground ginger
- 1/4 tsp of salt
- 1/4 tsp of vanilla extract
- 1 tbsp [12g] of chia seeds
- 1/4 cup [60ml] of unsweetened almond milk

Directions:
1. Preheat the oven to 350°F [175°C].
2. In a bowl, combine the mashed sweet potato, almond flour, rolled oats, coconut oil, maple syrup, cinnamon, ginger, salt, and vanilla extract. Mix until fully incorporated.
3. Add the chia seeds and almond milk to the mixture and stir again. The mixture should be thick but pourable.
4. Line a small baking dish (8x8 inches or 20x20 cm) with parchment paper or lightly grease it.
5. Pour the sweet potato mixture into the prepared dish, spreading it evenly with a spatula.
6. Bake for 30-35 minutes, or until the bars are set and lightly golden on top.
7. Let the bars cool completely in the dish before slicing them into squares.

Pear and Quinoa Crumble

Time: 45 minutes	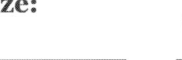 **Serving Size:** 2 servings
Prep Time: 15 minutes	**Cook Time:** 30 minutes

Each Serving Has:
Calories: 180, Carbohydrates: 35g, Saturated Fat: 3g, Protein: 4g, Fat: 6g, Sodium: 20mg, Potassium: 230mg, Fiber: 5g, Sugar: 18g, Vitamin C: 6mg, Calcium: 30mg, Iron: 1.2mg.

Ingredients:
- 2 medium pears, peeled, cored, and diced (about 2 cups) [300g]
- 1/4 cup [40g] of quinoa, rinsed
- 1/4 cup [24g] of rolled oats
- 1 tbsp [14g] of coconut oil, melted
- 1 tbsp [21g] of maple syrup
- 1/4 tsp of ground cinnamon
- 1/4 tsp of ground ginger
- 1 tbsp [12g] of chia seeds
- 1 tbsp [15ml] of unsweetened almond milk
- Pinch of salt

Directions:
1. Preheat the oven to 350°F [175°C].
2. Bring 1/2 cup of water to a boil in a saucepan. Add the rinsed quinoa, reduce the heat, and simmer for 10-12 minutes until tender and the water is absorbed. Remove from heat and set aside.
3. In a bowl, combine the pears, cinnamon, ginger, and maple syrup. Stir to coat the pears evenly.
4. In a separate bowl, mix the cooked quinoa, oats, melted coconut oil, chia seeds, almond milk, and a pinch of salt. This will form the crumble topping.
5. Transfer the seasoned pears to a small baking dish. Evenly distribute the quinoa-oat mixture on top of the pears.
6. Bake for 25-30 minutes, until the top is golden brown and the pears are tender.
7. Let the crumble cool for a few minutes before serving.

Baked Pear and Oat Tart

Time: 50 minutes	 **Serving Size:** 2 servings
Prep Time: 15 minutes	**Cook Time:** 35 minutes

Each Serving Has:
Calories: 236, Carbohydrates: 37g, Saturated Fat: 0.6g, Protein: 5g, Fat: 8g, Sodium: 42mg, Potassium: 295mg, Fiber: 5g, Sugar: 14g, Vitamin C: 5mg, Calcium: 58mg, Iron: 1.2mg

Ingredients:
- 1/2 cup [50g] rolled oats
- 1/4 cup [30g] oat flour
- 1 tbsp olive oil
- 1 tbsp maple syrup
- 1 tbsp unsweetened oat milk
- 1/4 tsp ground
- cinnamon
- 1/8 tsp sea salt (optional)
- 1 large pear, peeled, cored, and thinly sliced [about 150g]
- 1/2 tsp vanilla extract
- 1/2 tsp olive oil, for greasing

Directions:
1. Preheat the oven to 350°F [175°C]. Lightly grease a 5-inch tart pan or small oven-safe dish with olive oil.
2. In a medium bowl, combine rolled oats, oat flour, olive oil, maple syrup, unsweetened oat milk, ground cinnamon, and sea salt (if using). Mix until the dough holds together.
3. Press the oat mixture evenly into the prepared tart pan, forming a crust along the bottom and up the sides slightly.
4. Arrange thinly sliced pear in overlapping layers on top of the crust.
5. Drizzle the vanilla extract evenly over the pear slices.
6. Bake for 35 minutes, until the pears are tender and the crust is lightly golden.
7. Allow the tart to cool for 10 minutes before slicing and serving warm.

Steamed Pear Pudding with Maple Syrup

 Time:
40 minutes

 Serving Size:
2 servings

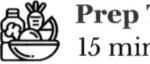 **Prep Time:**
15 minutes

 Cook Time:
25 minutes

Each Serving Has:

Calories: 210, Carbohydrates: 52g, Saturated Fat: 1g, Protein: 2g, Fat: 3g, Sodium: 25mg, Potassium: 320mg, Fiber: 6g, Sugar: 35g, Vitamin C: 12mg, Calcium: 40mg, Iron: 0.5mg.

Ingredients:

- 1/2 cup [90g] of rinsed millet
- 1 1/2 cups [360ml] of unsweetened oat milk
- 1 tbsp of chopped soft dates
- 1/2 tsp of ground cinnamon
- 1/2 tsp of vanilla extract
- 1 tsp of olive oil
- 2 medium pears, peeled, cored, and diced
- 2 tbsp of water
- 1 tbsp of maple syrup

Directions:

1. In a bowl, combine the whole wheat flour, oats, cinnamon, ginger, flaxseed, and a pinch of salt. Stir to mix evenly.
2. Add the pears to the dry mixture and toss gently to coat.
3. In a separate bowl, whisk together the almond milk, maple syrup, melted coconut oil, and vanilla extract.
4. Pour the wet mixture over the pear and dry ingredients and stir gently until everything is well combined.
5. Lightly grease ramekins with coconut oil. Divide the pear mixture between them, pressing gently to compact.
6. Place a steamer basket over boiling water, making sure it doesn't touch the ramekins. Cover and steam for 25 minutes, until set and cooked through.
7. Remove the ramekins from the steamer and cool before serving.

Pumpkin Spice Oat Balls

 Time:
15 minutes

 Serving Size:
2 balls

 Prep Time:
10 minutes

 Cook Time:
5 minutes

Each Serving Has:

Calories: 180, Carbohydrates: 28g, Saturated Fat: 1g, Protein: 4g, Fat: 7g, Sodium: 60mg, Potassium: 160mg, Fiber: 4g, Sugar: 7g, Vitamin C: 3mg, Calcium: 35mg, Iron: 1mg.

Ingredients:

- 1/2 cup [40g] of rolled oats
- 1/4 cup [60g] of canned pumpkin puree
- 2 tbsp [30g] of almond butter
- 1 tbsp [15ml] of maple syrup
- 1/2 tsp of ground
- cinnamon
- 1/4 tsp of ground ginger
- 1/4 tsp of ground nutmeg
- 1 tbsp [7g] of ground flaxseed
- Pinch of salt
- 1 tsp of vanilla extract

Directions:

1. In a mixing bowl, combine the oats, pumpkin puree, almond butter, maple syrup, cinnamon, ginger, nutmeg, flaxseed, and a pinch of salt.
2. Stir the mixture together until well combined. If the mixture is too sticky, add a little extra oats or flaxseed to help with the consistency.
3. Add the vanilla extract and mix again until evenly distributed.
4. Once the mixture is fully incorporated, use your hands to shape it into small balls, about 1 inch in diameter. You should be able to make about 8 balls.
5. Place the balls on a parchment-lined tray or plate and refrigerate for 5 minutes to firm them up.
6. Serve chilled or at room temperature.

Baked Rice and Apple Pudding

 Time:
45 minutes

 Serving Size:
2 servings

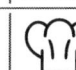 **Prep Time:**
10 minutes

 Cook Time:
35 minutes

Each Serving Has:
Calories: 250, Carbohydrates: 50g, Saturated Fat: 1g, Protein: 4g, Fat: 3g, Sodium: 55mg, Potassium: 220mg, Fiber: 4g, Sugar: 18g, Vitamin C: 5mg, Calcium: 50mg, Iron: 1mg.

Ingredients:
- 1/2 cup [85g] of cooked white rice
- 1 medium apple, peeled and diced [150g]
- 1/2 cup [120ml] of almond milk
- 2 tbsp [30g] of honey
- 1/4 tsp of ground cinnamon
- 1/4 tsp of ground nutmeg
- 1 large egg
- 1/2 tsp of vanilla extract
- 2 tbsp [14g] of ground flaxseed
- 1 tbsp [15g] of coconut oil, melted

Directions:
1. Preheat the oven to 350°F [175°C] and grease a small baking dish with coconut oil.
2. In a bowl, combine the cooked rice, apple, almond milk, honey, cinnamon, and nutmeg. Stir until well mixed.
3. In a separate bowl, beat the egg with the vanilla extract and flaxseed until smooth.
4. Add the egg mixture to the rice and apple mixture, and stir to combine.
5. Pour the mixture into the prepared baking dish and smooth it out with a spatula.
6. Drizzle the melted coconut oil over the top and bake in the preheated oven for 30-35 minutes, or until the top is golden and set.
7. Remove from the oven and let it cool slightly before serving.

Pumpkin and Rice Pudding Squares

 Time:
1 hour

Serving Size:
2 servings

 Prep Time:
15 minutes

Cook Time:
45 minutes

Each Serving Has:
Calories: 214, Carbohydrates: 36g, Saturated Fat: 0.6g, Protein: 4g, Fat: 6g, Sodium: 28mg, Potassium: 258mg, Fiber: 3g, Sugar: 10g, Vitamin C: 5mg, Calcium: 56mg, Iron: 1.3mg

Ingredients:
- 1/2 cup [100g] cooked short-grain brown rice, cooled
- 1/2 cup [120g] mashed steamed pumpkin
- 1/2 cup [120ml] unsweetened oat milk
- 2 tbsp maple
- syrup
- 1 tbsp ground flaxseed
- 1/4 cup [25g] quick oats
- 1/2 tsp ground cinnamon
- 1/2 tsp vanilla extract
- 1/2 tsp olive oil

Directions:
1. Preheat the oven to 350°F [175°C]. Lightly grease a small square baking dish (about 5×5 inches) with olive oil.
2. In a large bowl, combine cooked brown rice, mashed pumpkin, oat milk, maple syrup, ground flaxseed, quick oats, ground cinnamon, and vanilla extract. Stir well to form a smooth, thick mixture.
3. Pour the mixture into the prepared baking dish and smooth the top with a spatula.
4. Bake for 45 minutes, until the edges are set and lightly golden and the center is firm to the touch.
5. Allow to cool in the dish for 10 minutes before slicing into squares. Serve warm.

Quinoa Flaxseed Bars with Apple

 Time:
50 minutes

 Serving Size:
2 servings

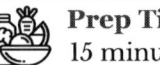 **Prep Time:**
15 minutes

Cook Time:
35 minutes

Each Serving Has:
Calories: 218, Carbohydrates: 34g, Saturated Fat: 0.6g, Protein: 5g, Fat: 7g, Sodium: 23mg, Potassium: 298mg, Fiber: 5g, Sugar: 11g, Vitamin C: 6mg, Calcium: 52mg, Iron: 1.4mg

Ingredients:
- 1/2 cup [85g] rinsed quinoa
- 1 cup [240ml] water
- 1 tbsp ground flaxseed
- 1 tbsp maple syrup
- 1/4 tsp ground cinnamon
- 1/2 tsp vanilla extract
- 1/2 cup [120g] peeled, cored, and diced apple
- 1/4 cup [25g] quick oats
- 1 tsp olive oil

Directions:
1. Preheat the oven to 350°F [175°C]. Grease a loaf pan with olive oil.
2. Combine quinoa and water in a medium saucepan. Bring to a boil, then reduce to low, cover, and simmer for 15 minutes until tender and water is absorbed. Let sit covered, then fluff with a fork and cool slightly.
3. Place the diced apple in a small steamer basket over simmering water. Cover and steam for 10 minutes, until the apple is soft. Remove from heat and let it cool slightly.
4. In a bowl, combine cooked quinoa, ground flaxseed, maple syrup, cinnamon, vanilla extract, oats, and steamed apple. Stir until thick and cohesive.
5. Press the mixture firmly into the loaf pan, smoothing the top.
6. Bake for 20 minutes, until the edges are golden and the center is firm.
7. Cool completely in the pan before slicing into bars, then serve.

Blueberry and Chia Yogurt Bowls

 Time:
10 minutes

 Serving Size:
2 bowls

 Prep Time:
10 minutes

 Cook Time:
0 minutes

Each Serving Has:
Calories: 180, Carbohydrates: 26g, Saturated Fat: 1g, Protein: 9g, Fat: 7g, Sodium: 60mg, Potassium: 200mg, Fiber: 6g, Sugar: 14g, Vitamin C: 8mg, Calcium: 100mg, Iron: 0.7mg.

Ingredients:
- 1 cup [240ml] of plain Greek yogurt
- 1/4 cup [40g] of chia seeds
- 1/2 cup [75g] of blueberries
- 1 tbsp [15ml] of maple syrup
- 1/4 tsp of vanilla extract
- 1/4 cup [60ml] of unsweetened almond milk
- 1 tbsp [8g] of sliced almonds (optional)

Directions:
1. In a bowl, combine the Greek yogurt, chia seeds, maple syrup, and vanilla extract. Stir well to ensure the chia seeds are evenly distributed throughout the yogurt.
2. Add the almond milk to the yogurt mixture, and stir again until the mixture reaches your desired consistency. The almond milk helps to thin the mixture slightly while keeping it creamy.
3. Refrigerate the yogurt mixture for at least 2 hours (or overnight) to allow the chia seeds to expand and create a pudding-like consistency.
4. Once ready to serve, top each bowl with fresh blueberries and a sprinkle of sliced almonds (if using).

Carrot and Cinnamon Bars

 Time:
30 minutes

 Serving Size:
2 bars

 Prep Time:
10 minutes

Cook Time:
20 minutes

Each Serving Has:

Calories: 170, Carbohydrates: 30g, Saturated Fat: 2g, Protein: 3g, Fat: 6g, Sodium: 90mg, Potassium: 300mg, Fiber: 5g, Sugar: 12g, Vitamin C: 3mg, Calcium: 40mg, Iron: 1mg.

Ingredients:

- 1 cup [120g] of grated carrots
- 1/2 cup [45g] of rolled oats
- 1/4 cup [60ml] of unsweetened applesauce
- 1/4 cup [30g] of almond flour
- 1/2 tsp of ground cinnamon
- 1/4 tsp of baking soda
- 1/8 tsp of salt
- 1/4 cup [60ml] of maple syrup
- 1/4 cup [60ml] of unsweetened almond milk
- 1 tsp of vanilla extract

Directions:

1. Preheat your oven to 350°F [175°C].
2. In a bowl, combine the carrots, oats, almond flour, cinnamon, baking soda, and salt. Stir well to combine.
3. In a separate bowl, whisk together the maple syrup, almond milk, and vanilla extract until fully combined.
4. Pour the wet ingredients into the dry ingredients and stir until well combined.
5. Line a small baking pan (approximately 8x8 inches or 20x20 cm) with parchment paper. Pour the mixture into the pan and spread it evenly.
6. Bake for 20 minutes, or until a toothpick inserted into the center comes out clean.
7. Let the bars cool in the pan for about 10 minutes before transferring to a wire rack to cool completely.
8. Slice into squares and serve.

Low-Fat Peach Tartlets

 Time:
45 minutes

 Serving Size:
2 tartlets

 Prep Time:
15 minutes

 Cook Time:
30 minutes

Each Serving Has:

Calories: 160, Carbohydrates: 36g, Saturated Fat: 1g, Protein: 3g, Fat: 3g, Sodium: 30mg, Potassium: 200mg, Fiber: 4g, Sugar: 25g, Vitamin C: 6mg, Calcium: 20mg, Iron: 1mg.

Ingredients:

- 1 cup [150g] of fresh peaches, peeled and sliced
- 1/4 cup [30g] of whole wheat flour
- 1/4 cup [30g] of almond flour
- 2 tbsp [30g] of honey
- 2 tbsp [30ml] of unsweetened applesauce
- 1/4 tsp of ground cinnamon
- 1/2 tsp of vanilla extract
- 1/8 tsp of salt
- 1 tbsp [12g] of chia seeds
- 1 tbsp [15ml] of water

Directions:

1. Preheat your oven to 350°F [175°C].
2. In a bowl, combine the chia seeds with the water and let them sit for about 5 minutes to form a gel.
3. In a separate bowl, mix together the whole wheat flour, almond flour, cinnamon, and salt. Add the honey, applesauce, and vanilla extract to the dry ingredients. Stir well until the mixture forms a dough.
4. Divide the dough into two portions and press each into a tartlet pan, smoothing the edges to form a crust.
5. Combine peaches and chia seed gel in a saucepan. Heat gently over low for about 5 minutes to soften the peaches.
6. Spoon the peach mixture evenly into the prepared tartlet crusts.
7. Bake the tartlets for about 20-30 minutes or until the crusts are golden.
8. Remove the tartlets from the oven and cool for 10 minutes before serving.

Papaya and Almond Butter Mousse

Time: 15 minutes	**Serving Size:** 2 small bowls
Prep Time: 10 minutes	**Cook Time:** 5 minutes

Each Serving Has:

Calories: 180, Carbohydrates: 25g, Saturated Fat: 2g, Protein: 3g, Fat: 9g, Sodium: 10mg, Potassium: 350mg, Fiber: 4g, Sugar: 15g, Vitamin C: 40mg, Calcium: 40mg, Iron: 1mg.

Ingredients:

- 1 ripe papaya, peeled and chopped [200g]
- 2 tbsp [30g] of almond butter
- 1 tbsp [21g] of honey
- 1/2 tsp of vanilla extract
- 1/4 tsp of ground cinnamon
- 1 tbsp [12g] of chia seeds
- 1 tbsp [15ml] of water

Directions:

1. Prepare the chia seeds by combining them with water in a small bowl. Stir well and let the mixture sit for about 5 minutes, until it thickens into a gel-like consistency.
2. While the chia seeds are setting, prepare the papaya by peeling and chopping it into small chunks.
3. Place the papaya, almond butter, honey, vanilla extract, and cinnamon into a blender or food processor. Blend until the mixture is smooth and creamy.
4. Add the chia seed gel to the blender and blend again until fully incorporated into the mousse.
5. Transfer the mousse to small serving dishes, cover, and refrigerate for 1 hour to chill and thicken.
6. Serve the mousse chilled, garnished with a sprinkle of cinnamon or a few extra chia seeds if desired.

Chapter 8: 28-Day Meal Prep Plan

Week	Day	Breakfast	Lunch	Snack or appetizer	Dinner
Week 1:	1	Chickpea Flour Pancakes with Fresh Herbs	Chicken Millet Patties with Dill Yogurt	Roasted Fennel Slices	White Fish with Zucchini and Quinoa
	2	Buckwheat and Apple Flatbread	Lentil and Roasted Fennel Casserole	Pumpkin Seed and Flax Energy Bars	Vegetables with Wild Rice and Fennel
	3	Baked Millet Cakes with Pear and Cardamom	Zucchini Noodles with Basil Pesto	Soft Baked Pear and Oat Bars	Steamed Halibut with Parsley and Wild Rice
	4	Banana and Oat Breakfast Cookies	Shrimp Rice Noodles with Zucchini	Baked Zucchini Sticks with Basil Yogurt Dip	Sweet Potato and Fennel Gratin
	5	Polenta with Steamed Pears	Baked Turkey Patties with Sweet Potato Mash	Chia Coconut Cups with Poached Apple	Turkey Breast with Millet and Pumpkin Puree
	6	Amaranth Porridge with Vanilla and Blueberries	Creamy Broccoli and Rice Soup	Roasted Cauliflower Bites with Garlic-Free Sauce	Lentil and Cauliflower Casserole
	7	Rice Porridge with Banana and Cinnamon	Butternut Squash and Quinoa Pilaf with Dill	Apple and Cinnamon Snack Bites	Roasted Pumpkin and Mushroom Bowl
Week 2:	8	Chickpea Flour Pancakes with Fresh Herbs	Steamed Halibut with Dill Rice and Tender Chayote	Carrot and Zucchini Muffins	Cauliflower and Spinach Bake
	9	Roasted Carrot and Oat Porridge	Steamed Cod with Carrot Puree and Quinoa	Steamed Green Beans with Herb Dressing	Lentil and Cabbage Stew with Sweet Potatoes
	10	Buckwheat and Banana Muffins	Broccoli and Sweet Potato Grain Bowl	Rice Cakes with Pumpkin Spread	Barley Pilaf with Roasted Carrots
	11	Sweet Potato and Spinach Breakfast Bowl	Chicken Strips with Wild Rice and Green Beans	Roasted Chickpeas with Dill and Olive Oil	Poached Chicken with Asparagus and Parsley
	12	Soft Polenta with Pumpkin Puree	Roasted Carrot and Barley Salad	Cucumber and Spinach Pinwheels	Herb-Roasted Vegetables with Brown Rice
	13	Zucchini and Herb Scramble	Lentil and Sweet Potato Salad with Parsley	Wild Rice and Cucumber Salad Cups	Quinoa and Roasted Pumpkin Bowl
	14	Buckwheat and Coconut Milk Porridge with Pears	Pumpkin Stew with Barley	Baked Carrot and Quinoa Balls	Shrimp with Rice Noodles and Bok Choy

Week	Day	Breakfast	Lunch	Snack or appetizer	Dinner
Week 3:	15	Applesauce Pancakes with Chia Seeds	Baked Bell Peppers with Quinoa	Kohlrabi Sticks with Yogurt Dip	Lentil and Wild Rice Casserole
	16	Soft Oatmeal Pancakes with Blueberries	Cauliflower and Zucchini Casserole	Baked Plantain Chips with Sea Salt	Fish Fillets with Steamed Green Beans
	17	Spinach and Asparagus Egg Wraps	Braised Vegetables with Quinoa	Roasted Beet Chips with Olive Oil	Baked Chicken with Herb Sauce
	18	Baked Apple Quinoa Casserole	Quinoa and Broccoli Bowl with Olive Oil	White Bean and Basil Dip with Rice Crackers	Wild Rice and Mushroom Casserole
	19	Rice Flake Cereal with Almond Milk	Roasted Beetroot and Cauliflower Bowl	Polenta Squares with Roasted Sunchokes and Parsnips	Pumpkin and Chickpea Stew
	20	Banana and Oat Breakfast Cookies	Poached White Fish with Steamed Vegetables	Carrot and Celery Sticks with Yogurt Dill Dip	Rice and Zucchini Casserole with Soft Tofu
	21	Barley and Apple Breakfast Cereal	Turkey and Millet Stuffed Cabbage Rolls	Steamed Edamame with Parsley	Roasted Carrot and Fennel Bake
Week 4:	22	Quinoa and Poppy Seed Breakfast Bars	Roasted Pumpkin and Fennel Bowl	Apple and Cinnamon Snack Bites	White Fish with Barley and Carrot Puree
	23	Millet and Pumpkin Breakfast Bowl	Creamy Lentil and Spinach Soup	Soft Baked Pear and Oat Bars	Millet and Spinach Bake with Dill Sauce
	24	Chickpea Flour Pancakes with Fresh Herbs	Wild Rice and Mushroom Bowl with Parsley	Steamed Carrot and Wild Rice Salad	Baked Sweet Bell Peppers with Millet and Herbs
	25	Buckwheat and Apple Flatbread	Quinoa and Cucumber Salad with Fresh Dill	Roasted Parsnip Sticks with Thyme	Roasted Pumpkin and Mushroom Bowl
	26	Amaranth Porridge with Vanilla and Blueberries	Green Bean and Buckwheat Salad	Chia Coconut Cups with Poached Apple	Lentil and Cauliflower Casserole
	27	Zucchini and Sweet Potato Breakfast Hash	Low-Acid Pumpkin Soup with Parsley	Rice Paper Rolls	Poached Chicken with Asparagus and Parsley
	28	Pumpkin Spice Oatmeal with Maple Syrup	Carrot, Fennel, and Quinoa Warm Salad	Baked Zucchini Sticks with Basil Yogurt Dip	Chicken Thighs with Barley and Carrots

Free Gift

Thank you! Discover your gift inside! Dive into a rich assortment of DASH Diet for Beginners recipes for added inspiration. Gift it or share the PDF effortlessly with friends and family via a single click on WhatsApp or other social platforms. Bon appétit!

Conclusion outline

As you turn the final pages of this cookbook, take a moment to recognize the progress you've made. You began this journey seeking relief, clarity, and a way to enjoy food again without discomfort — and now you have a powerful set of tools at your fingertips.

Throughout these chapters, you've learned more than just how to avoid reflux triggers. You've discovered how to nourish your body with intention, using simple, accessible ingredients and practical cooking methods that fit your real life. Whether you're brand new to the kitchen or simply looking for less complicated ways to eat well, I hope these recipes have shown you that eating for acid reflux doesn't have to be restrictive, bland, or stressful.

It's important to remember that no two bodies are exactly the same. While this book offers a strong foundation based on common reflux-safe principles, your personal experience will guide you further. Pay attention to how your body responds, and don't be afraid to adjust recipes or routines to suit your needs. Flexibility is not a sign of failure — it's a mark of strength and self-awareness.

Most of all, I hope you walk away from this book feeling empowered. You now have the knowledge to take control of your symptoms, the confidence to cook nourishing meals, and the reassurance that food can once again be a source of comfort, not worry.

Healing is not about perfection — it's about progress. Keep moving forward, one thoughtful meal at a time. You deserve to feel good in your body, and you have everything you need to begin.

Here's to comfort, clarity, and the joy of eating well.

References

Altomare, D. F., Portincasa, P., & Palasciano, G. (2013). Gastroesophageal reflux disease (GERD): Pathophysiology and treatment options. Clinical Gastroenterology, 27(2), 89–95. https://doi.org/10.1016/j.clinre.2013.01.006

Katz, P. O., Gerson, L. B., & Vela, M. F. (2013). Guidelines for the diagnosis and management of gastroesophageal reflux disease. The American Journal of Gastroenterology, 108(3), 308–328. https://doi.org/10.1038/ajg.2012.444

National Institute of Diabetes and Digestive and Kidney Diseases. (2022). Gastroesophageal reflux (GER) and gastroesophageal reflux disease (GERD). U.S. Department of Health and Human Services. https://www.niddk.nih.gov/health-information/digestive-diseases/acid-reflux-ger-gerd-adults

Pellegrini, C. A. (2020). Dietary and lifestyle modifications in GERD patients. In Y. Hashash & W. A. Faubion Jr. (Eds.), Nutrition in gastrointestinal disease (pp. 115–126). Springer. https://doi.org/10.1007/978-3-030-30345-4_9

Westbrook, J., & Davidson, C. (2019). The GERD & Acid Reflux Solution: A Cookbook and Lifestyle Guide for Healing Heartburn Naturally. Harmony Wellness Press.

Zalvan, C. H., Hu, S., Greenberg, B., & Geliebter, J. (2017). A comparison of alkaline water and Mediterranean-style diet vs. proton pump inhibition for laryngopharyngeal reflux. JAMA Otolaryngology–Head & Neck Surgery, 143(10), 1023–1029. https://doi.org/10.1001/jamaoto.2017.1454

Zibdeh, R. (2020). The acid reflux diet cookbook for beginners: A 3-week meal plan and 100 simple recipes to restore digestive health. Rockridge Press.

DeVault, K. R. (2016). The complete acid reflux diet plan: Easy meal plans and recipes to heal GERD and LPR. Rockridge Press.

Martinson, S. (2019). Dropping acid: The reflux diet cookbook & cure. Reflux Cookbooks.

Koufman, J. A., & Stern, S. R. (2011). Dropping acid: The reflux diet cookbook & cure. Katalitix Media.

Appendix 1: Measurement Conversion Chart

U.S. System	Metric
1 inch	2.54 centimeters
1 fluid ounce	29.57 milliliters
1 pint (16 ounces)	473.18 milliliters, 2 cups
1 quart (32 ounces)	1 liter, 4 cups
1 gallon (128 ounces)	4 liters, 16 cups
1 pound (16 ounces)	437.5 grams (0.4536 kilogram), 473.18 milliliters
1 ounces	2 tablespoons, 28 grams
1 cup (8 ounces)	237 milliliters
1 teaspoon	5 milliliters
1 tablespoon	15 milliliters (3 teaspoons)
Fahrenheit (subtract 32 and divide by 1.8 to get Celsius)	Centigrade (multiply by 1.8 and add 32 to get Fahrenheit)

Appendix 2: Index Recipes

Notes